We Miss You All

Noerine Kaleeba: AIDS in the Family

Noerine Kaleeba with Sunanda Ray and Brigid Willmore

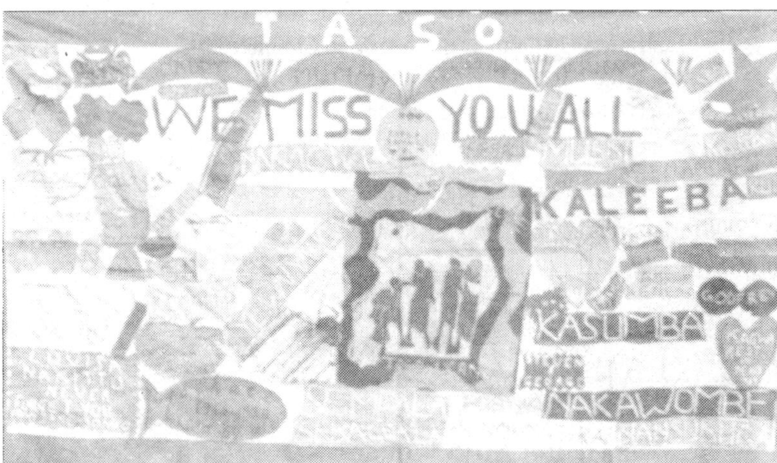

Women and AIDS Support Network (WASN), Zimbabwe

Illustrations and cover design: Jane Shepherd
Title page photograph: Tessa Colvin
Typesetting: Brigid Willmore

ISBN: 0 7974 1009 0

We Miss You All is published by the
Women and AIDS Support Network (WASN)
P O Box 1554, Harare, Zimbabwe

with the financial and moral support of the
Swedish International Development Authority (SIDA)
Harare, Zimbabwe

We Miss You All

Contents

Dedication

I would like to dedicate this book to five women:

My four daughters Elizabeth, Phiona, Marion and Christine for whom it is my heart's desire that this book forms a basis for their protection against AIDS

and

My mother in law, Zabeeti, who silently mourns the death of her children, but has been a source of encouragement to me. A grandmother with an ever increasing number of orphaned grandchildren.

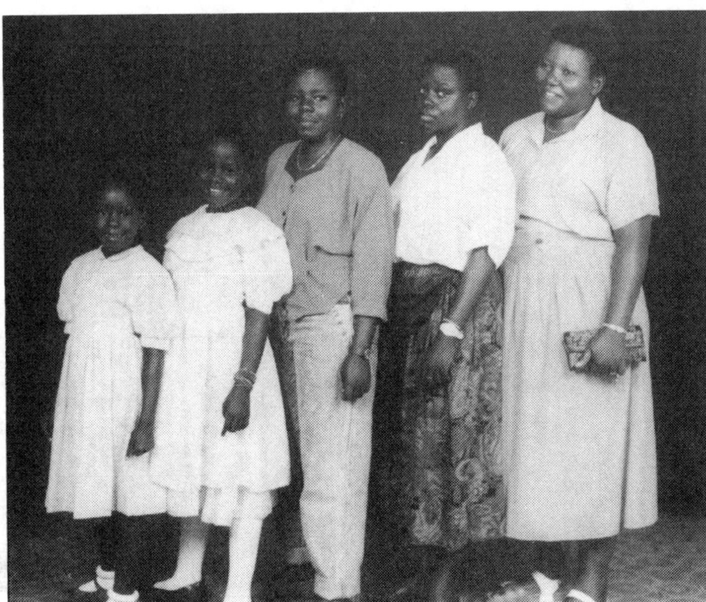

We would like to thank a number of people who have assisted with the production of **We Miss You All**:

Mary Bassett, Eileen Chinyadza, Rachel Howard, Helen Jackson, Mercy Jumo, Farai Madzimbamuto, Tambudzai Madzimbamuto, Sarah Laher, Constance Samuwi, AnneLorne Thwaites, and Everjoyce Win.

Thanks must also be extended to SIDA, the Swedish International Development Authority, for their support; and to the National AIDS Control Programme (NACP) Zimbabwe for their endorsement of the project.

Noerine Kaleeba, Sunanda Ray and Brigid Willmore

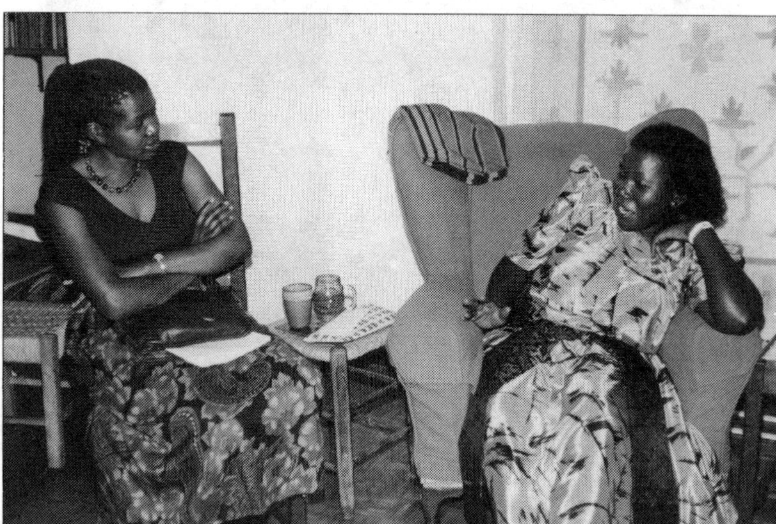

Noerine and Constance (Secretary, WASN)

Acknowledgements

I thank all my friends, a long inexhaustible list. A few will appear in this account, others I met only briefly, many are no longer in this world, but all have made a permanent impression on my life.

But particularly I want to thank:

My closest friends, my four daughters: Elizabeth, Phiona, Marion, and Christine

My dear late husband, Christopher (rest in loving peace)

My parents and parents-in-law

My late father, Tadeo Lutwaama (rest in loving peace)

The staff, doctors and nurses at Castle Hill Hospital: Dr Nanda, Sister Wulthers, Sister Camilla Fisher, Nurse Pat Chew, Janet, Ann, Dr Symonds, and Father Storey

My friends at the British Council: Debbi Vowels, Jan Webster, Norma Branton, and Keith Bintl

My friends at work: Mary, Peter, Florence, Margaret, Clare, Fred

My friends with whom we started and developed TASO: David, Nastor, Mary, Jason, Rose, Jane, Charles, Godfrey, Peter, Wilson, Winifred, Rachael, Deborah, Musa, Nampologoma, Joyce, Colin, Joseph, Juma, Betty, Henry, Molly, Kate.

A long long list.

Now I thank God for my two newly found friends who are willing to help me to share my life with other people. Thanks to you Sunanda and Brigid, what I have experienced, what I feel, how I have gone about life, may benefit other people going through similar experiences. I have always felt that this might be useful to people but I have never felt capable of writing it down in an organised way. I also thank you Sunanda for your insistence, which has helped me to deal with the inertia of getting started. I also want to say that the task you two are taking on is great, sorting out the mess of events, ideas and emotions expressed by me and presenting them in a useful manner.

I will write this account of my life and my continuing encounter with AIDS as honestly and accurately as I can. I will not attempt to give excuses, even where they exist, but will give a straight account and rely on your understanding and friendship to deal with issues sensitively. Our goal is to produce a book which will support other people in my situation.

Thank you all.

Noerine Kaleeba

Preface

As I begin this long account of my life and the circumstances surrounding my personal encounter with AIDS, I want to thank God and offer glory to His Name for the three special gifts he has given me:

The Gift of Life
The Gift of My Four Children
The Gift of Friends.

I want every line of this account to be a reflection of my praise to God for his continued sustenance to me and my children, and a reflection of my gratitude to all my friends, to all people with AIDS, and to all those people who in one way or another have given friendship, true friendship, to people with HIV and AIDS.

This morning I went to church in Harare, at the Cathedral of the Sacred Heart. By coincidence, the special thought for the day was *A Friend is a Gift of God.* It says:

"Among the great glorious gifts our heavenly Father sends is
the gift of understanding that we find in loving friends
For in this world of trouble that is filled with anxious care
Everybody needs a friend in whom they are free to share
The little secret heartaches that lay heavy on their mind
Not just a mere acquaintance but someone who's Just Our Kind
For somehow in the generous heart of loving faithful friends
The good God in his charity and wisdom always sends
A sense of understanding and the power of perception
And mixes these the parent of all other virtues."

Noerine Kaleeba
Harare, September 1990

AIDS came to my house on the afternoon of the 6th June 1986, when the British Council sent me a telex to tell me that my husband Chris was seriously ill in a hospital in England. He had gone to Hull University to do his postgraduate training the previous year.

I often wonder what my life would have been like today if that telex hadn't come. I know now that Chris was already very ill and dying, long before the telex was sent, but I always connect my misery and subsequent suffering to that telex. The British Council in Uganda did not know where I lived, but they knew from the papers Chris had filled in before he went to England that I worked at the School of Physiotherapy at Mulago, Kampala. Debbie Vowels, who was then working with the British Council in Kampala, first went to the School and found that I had just left to go to my parttime work with the Katalemwa Cheshire Home. In Uganda nearly everyone has more than one job, to make ends meet. At the Home she found that I had taken a group of disabled people to a meeting. As it was late she was given my home address, and went to a lot of trouble to find the house. She left an urgent message asking me to go the British Council Office the next morning. When I read the note I couldn't think what could have happened, but I knew immediately that it had to do with Chris.

The Fateful Telex

During our last telephone conversation in May Chris had told me that he was not coming home, as we had been so anxiously expecting. His request to register for a PhD had been accepted by the British Council, and so he would be away for another year. The girls were more disappointed than I was. They had already started crossing the days off on the calendar. I knew, however, he would be better off coming home with both a Masters degree and a PhD. The political atmosphere in Uganda was also getting better, and there was a general feeling of euphoria, so the prospect of another year without him was not as desperate as it would have been a year before.

Throughout that night in June, after receiving the message left for me by the British Council, I went through the possibilities. It never crossed my mind that Chris may be ill. So when I went into the British Council the next morning, and was given the telex, I was shocked. The message was clear and concise. My husband was critically ill in a British hospital. He had been unconscious for three days. Had he been involved in an accident again? No. He seemed to have meningitis. He was not in pain, but his condition was critical. Everything was being done for him. The British Council staff were very solicitous, offering tea, and comforting me. They suggested I return the next day for more news.

I left, walking like a zombie. Fortunately, I had come with my friend Mary, otherwise I would have been run over on the road. The following day I went back with my friends Margaret and Mary to the same news. His condition was still critical, everything that could be done was being done. Everyone was excessively nice and kind. I began to suspect that he had already died, and then to panic and make a scene. I wanted to go to him. He needed me. The Council people had to ask London first.

I went to a friend in the microbiology laboratory to ask him what he knew about meningitis. He suggested that I found out what type of meningitis Chris had. I went back to the British Council with the question. The following day the answer came, cryptococcal meningitis. My microbiology friend reacted in a funny way, and asked me if I was quite sure that it was cryptococcal.

I went back to the British Council and asked Debbie to write it down for me. My friend in the laboratory then asked me to find out if they had done an AIDS test. I vaguely wondered what the AIDS test had to do with it, but I went back the next day and asked the question. Everybody looked at each other. They said they would relay the question, and asked me to come back the next day to talk to the doctor on the phone. I can't quite recall how I got through those days, but I remember that the days merged into nights and I was crying a lot. The girls were devastated by my tears, and I couldn't even support them. All I knew was that Chris was dying. When I went back the next day, Dr Symonds told me on the phone that the AIDS test had been done, and it was positive. The news did not register right away. I was already saturated with misery. I did not believe it. There was no reason whatsoever to associate my husband with a white homosexual disease, which was what we knew about it in Uganda at that time.

I did not believe it, and I did not know the magnitude of the stigma associated with AIDS, so I told my friends at work and the neighbours. I told my in-laws, and my parents. I told anyone who came to sympathise with me.

Meanwhile arrangements were being made for me to go to Chris. I had to organise care for the children, so one of my sisters came to stay with them. The children suffered tremendously throughout this time. I was so locked up in my own selfpity and devastation that I did not know how to comfort them. During all this time, however, I was acutely aware of the kindness of the people at the British Council, although I was also aware that they were bewildered and seemed to know something they could not tell me.

My First Encounter with AIDS

In 1983 some doctors in Uganda had started reporting cases of a disease that seemed similar to one being reported in the USA. The reaction of the Ministry of Health was that we already had enough problems with the war and the poor state of the economy, without trying to deal with AIDS as well. Museveni, now President of Uganda, was in the bush then fighting the government, and things were really bad in the country. The attitude was: forget about AIDS, deal with the issues that you can do something about. After all, if people in the USA cannot cure AIDS then what is the point of saying we have AIDS too.

At the same time it was a sensitive issue, people were asking, where did this AIDS come from? Was it from America? Was it from Tanzania? At that time patients were being seen, but they were not talked about as having AIDS. Other words were used, like immunosuppression, because the instruction from the Ministry of Health was not to talk about AIDS, because this would create a scare which couldn't be dealt with then.

As a physiotherapist at Mulago Hospital I had heard intermittent reports of this mysterious and deadly illness, caused by a virus, that did not respond to treatment. The early reports connected the illness with white homosexual men in San Francisco, USA. At that time I had a few white friends who lived in Britain, but none of them were gay. Like many people my reaction was to dismiss the illness as having nothing to do with us in Uganda. But then, in the period 1983-84, we began to hear reports about a similar illness that was affecting people in the Kesensero area on the south west border with Tanzania. These people were associated with illicit trade across the border, which seemed to have something to do with the mysterious illness. There was also a strong rumour that the disease was highly infectious sexually and contagious. I still dismissed the problem, since there was nobody I knew in that area, nearly 200 kms from where I lived.

My very first encounter with a person with AIDS was very brief and promptly dismissed. Today the experience is very vivid in my mind.

I had gone to one of the medical wards in Mulago hospital to locate a paraplegic patient for a practical demonstration on the techniques of transferring a paraplegic from a bed to a wheelchair, for physiotherapy students. I located a young man who couldn't have been more than thirty years old. I introduced myself and explained what I required of him. He was very receptive and gave permission for my students to learn from him for that afternoon. His medical notes indicated that he had paraplegia due to Immunosuppression Syndrome, but I did not know what that was. I went to the ward sister to get permission to teach the students on her ward that afternoon, and to tell her which patient I had identified for the demonstration. She came closer to me and said "I wouldn't touch him if I were you. He has AIDS. We don't touch him, we only show his mother what to do".

I did not use him for the demonstration, neither did I go back to him to explain that I would not be coming. I cancelled the class and arranged for another patient from the orthopaedic ward.

I did not think about him again, until the diagnosis of AIDS came through my front door. Today there isn't a day which passes when I don't wonder what happened to him. With whom did he carry the burden? With whom did his mother carry the cross? What friends did she have to share her emotions? How much did he know about AIDS? What support did he have: God, children, loved ones? I suppose I will never know.

Meeting Chris

I was born at Seta Nazigo, a small village 35 kms southeast of Kampala, the third of ten children. I was educated at Sir Apollo School and Mount St Mary's Secondary School, a missionary boarding school run by Franciscan sisters. After my O levels I was accepted for training at the Mulago Hospital School of Physiotherapy.

I was in my third year at the School when I met Christopher. He was handsome and smart, about 25 years old, the same tribe as me, and he said he loved me. I had had other boyfriends before, one who was much older than I was and who used to give me many presents and spent a lot of money on me, but there had been no one I wanted to marry.

Chris had just graduated from the School of Radiography, and because he was ambitious he did not want children too soon. I found myself head over heels in love with him. Life with Christopher was different. Exciting. My first exposure to love. What I missed of the material things that my older friend had given me I made up for in love and companionship. I could show Christopher to my friends.

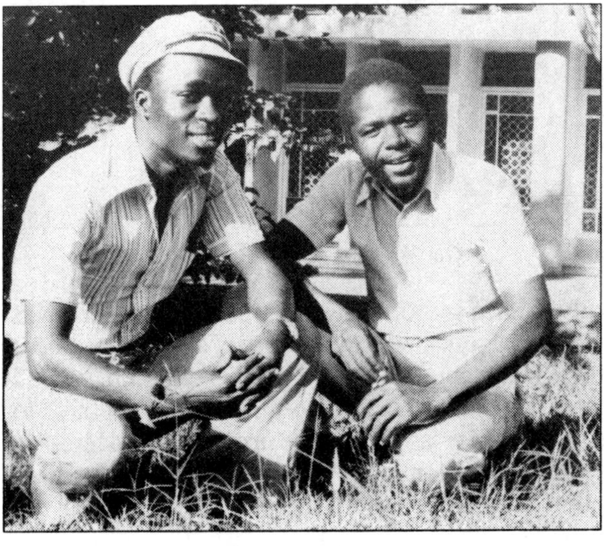

Chris (right) and friend

One of my early disappointments was that Chris was not accepted by my family. My father did not understand what I saw in this poor boy, and thought that because of his looks, he would not marry me but leave me high and dry as soon as he found another girlfriend. My mother's protests were even louder. Christopher was not a Catholic. My mother was always proud of having married a rich man, a chief, and having married in the Catholic Church. The situation was made worse because Chris and I lived together for a year and half, and had our first baby, Elizabeth, before we had saved enough money for the wedding. We had a modest Christmas wedding on the 27th December 1975, and our second daughter, Phiona, was born in April 1976.

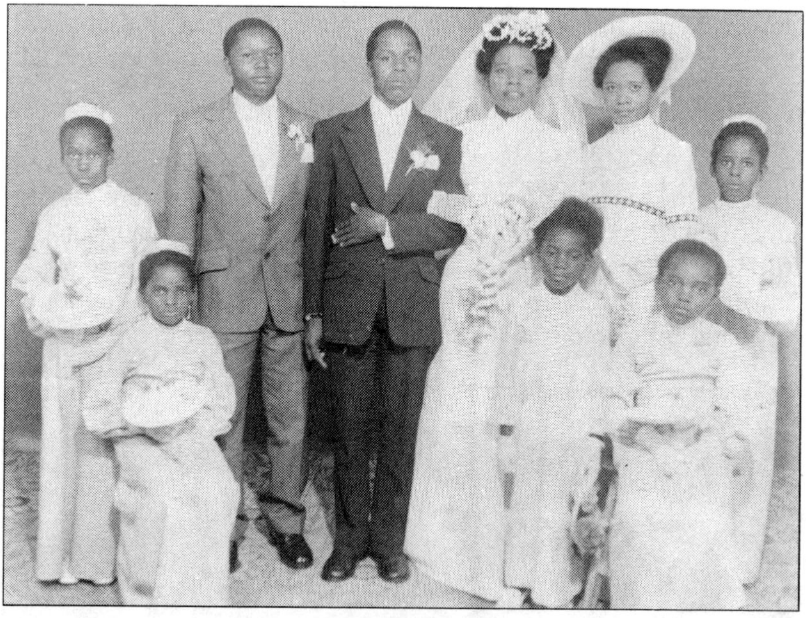

Our Wedding

Phiona was a lovely child, a carbon copy of her father, but Chris was disappointed not to have a son. It was even more of a disappointment for Chris because he had wanted to have only two children, while I had wanted six. Now that there were two girls, he would have to have a third child, a boy. This was a hard time in our relationship. We were struggling to make ends meet, and we had two very young children. I did not have any support from my parents, and my mother-in-law, who had been very supportive from a distance, was also disappointed that there was no son.

We quarrelled a bit with the first baby, and with the second, maybe even a little with the third. One of our problems was dealing with family planning and the need to limit pregnancy. We tried various family planning methods, including the condom. I did not fare well with the pill, and was scared to use an intrauterine device. So we used condoms, despite the fact that Chris did not like them much. He would use them, but became sulky afterwards and behaved as if he was unsatisfied.

Around this time Chris began a relationship with another woman, in search of a boy child. Although I suffered the stress of deprivation during this time, I did not feel betrayed, deserted, or angry at the other woman, because polygamy was something we had all grown up with. Another reason we didn't argue about the other woman was simply because our battles during that time were over the struggle to make ends meet, our resources were not enough. Our battles were not due to sexual jealousy, but over shortages in the house or the children going without something basic. Throughout this time Chris, because he loved me, did not behave in any way that showed that the other woman's presence divided his love.

The results of Chris' boy seeking ventures was another bonny little girl. She too was a carbon copy of her father, so much so that today when she and my Phiona stand side by side it is almost impossible to tell the difference between them. We rarely see her, but I hope she will one day want to join her sisters.

> I've thought about that hard time and our relationship a lot since then: about the arguments, about the other woman, about there never being enough money, the ups and downs of life. In early marriage it is difficult to cope. The babies come. They are always crying. You are tired from work. You have to prepare food. And then your husband goes out when he should be there to hold the baby while you cook. Our quarrels were about this, but the actual problems had stopped by the time Marion was born.

In the meantime, Chris had been studying privately for his A levels, and was accepted for a first degree at Makerere University. We were once again living happily as a family, and by the time Marion, our third child, was born in April 1980, we were a happy hardworking couple. I was working as a physiotherapy teacher, and Chris was studying sociology and social administration at Makerere. We suffered the life of married undergraduate students, but we were in love. Chris didn't seem to mind this time that Marion was a girl. Perhaps the shock of having tried for a boy elsewhere and having had a girl had taught him a lesson. We were maturing, and began to talk in a more constructive manner, began to plan for the future. I think that by this time we had made up our minds that we were going to remain together. You know when the first babies come, especially when you are still young, you think, from time to time, "One of these days maybe I'll divorce this man and find another one". But after the third baby we began to settle down.

In December 1980 I was awarded a British Council scholarship to study orthopaedic physiotherapy in the UK. I was away for 10 months, from January 1981. Chris was a wonderful father to the girls, who were still very young, and it was during this time that the tight bond between them was formed. This love, support and dependence on each other, was beautifully demonstrated during Chris' illness. The girls hold his memory as if he was still here.

When I returned to Uganda, and was appointed Principal of the School of Physiotherapy, Chris had graduated and was working as a teaching assistant in the Department of Adult Education at Makerere University. He had graduated with an honours degree, despite having been a single parent during the worst time of his examinations. We were now earning a little more, the children were at school, and we were very happy. Our fourth daughter was born on the 31st December 1983. We were still hoping for a boy, and had prepared to name him Christopher. As the baby turned out to be a girl we named her Christine, which was also appropriate since she was born at Christmas time.

Chris was making plans to go to England for further education. When the news came of his acceptance at Hull University, on a British Council scholarship, we were all overjoyed. He was very happy because he was finally going to realise his life's ambition to become a university professor. I was happy because he was happy, and the girls were happy because daddy was going to be a professor! If Chris returned with a PhD, it would mean a better job and a better way of life. I was also working hard. I had a parttime job with Cheshire Homes that brought in some extra money. I had also made a lot of friends. If Chris had returned in the way we hoped we would have had a good life.

Chris left for Hull in July 1985 to join the 1985/86 academic year, and registered for a Masters of Education in Sociology and Social Administration. His family were all there to see him off, together with the girls and I. I doubled my resolve to work hard and keep the girls in good shape for his return, just as he had done while I was away. This time the girls could also write to him. We were full of hope for the future.

We were not to know on that day at the airport that it would be the last time we would see him looking so tall, smart and handsome.

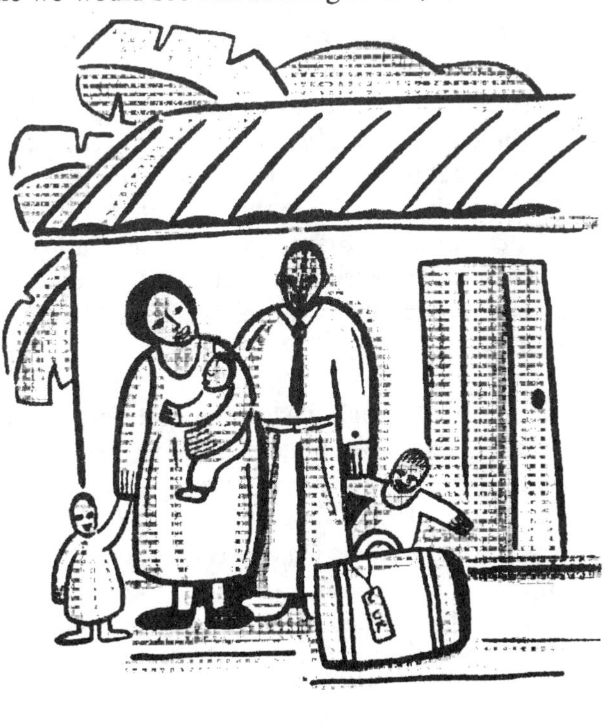

The War

After Chris left for England the girls and I settled down to the life of a family separated by distance but bound closely by the love they shared in letters and a telephone call once a month.

By about October 1985 Chris' letters began to contain complaints of stomach discomforts, unappetising food, and the total lack of any foodstuff that was appealing. I put this down to his inability to cook. In all the time I knew him he never cooked anything other than coffee or tea. I teased him about living in England and wanting to eat in Uganda.

By December 1985 the war that eventually brought the National Resistance Movement (NRM) lead by Museveni to power had reached a climax. Kampala was surrounded and mail was not moving. We talked to Chris on the phone, but the conversation was full of war news. The second week of January 1986, which saw Kampala fall to the NRA, was a nasty experience. I had to hide with the four girls in the basement of our flat, where we stayed with no food and little water for three days. The departing soldiers were molesting, stealing, and raping women as they went, and it was God's great mercy that by the time they came to our house we had already gone into hiding. After the fall of Kampala to the NRM, families with men were the first to get food, as remnants of the defeated army were still molesting women. I did not dare leave the girls on their own while I looked for food, and our first food came from the neighbours.

I missed Chris terribly through this experience. He, on the other hand, had his ears to the radio all the time for news of the war. He actually heard the news of the victory before we did.

I know now that during this time Chris was ill on and off with fever, loss of appetite, loss of weight, and mouth sores. He was also working doubly hard to complete his Masters degree and register for a PhD. His professor told me afterwards that he was working hard

> Five years ago in Uganda one man with a gun could walk through the door and take everything you had - just one man with one gun will make you lie down under the table and cover your face, while he takes everything. After you go through an experience like war, you come out a different person. Either you go down with the experience, or you rise, you are enhanced by the experience. So one of the things that the war experience has done for Ugandans is to produce a feeling of getting involved, a feeling of not wanting to suffer under the table.
> (WASN, 1990:19)

and did not look after himself well enough. He drank cupfuls of coffee and ate from a nearby fish and chip shop. Chris' explanation to himself for his ill health was that he was missing the staple Ugandan food (matooke), was working too hard, and was lonely and missing his family. On the 2nd June 1986 he was referred by the University Health Centre to Hull Royal Infirmary where he collapsed and was diagnosed as having cryptococcal meningitis (an infection of the brain specially linked to AIDS). He was transferred to the care of Dr Nanda at Castle Hill Hospital. It was there that the diagnosis of AIDS was made, when he was found to be HIV positive. In view of the grave diagnosis, and the fact that he was critically ill, the hospital asked the British Council to contact me in Uganda.

My Journey to Chris in England

I was finally able to leave Uganda to see Chris on the 12th June 1986. I hardly remember the journey which I seemed to make mechanically. I was met at Heathrow by a British Council guide, who took me to meet Jan Webster for the first time. Jan was then the Student Welfare Officer at the British Council in London, and was later to become a true and good family friend. Today she is one of the pillars of my support system. I was escorted on a three hour train journey to Hull, and on the afternoon of the 13th June 1986 I entered Ward 4 of Castle Hill Hospital, gently ushered into the staff room by Sister Camilla Fisher. After she offered me a cup of tea, which I could not drink, Dr Symonds, the house officer, came in to explain once more that Chris was gravely ill, that I would probably not recognise him, and that I needed to be very strong when I went into his room.

I heard all this and nodded as he explained, but my only thought was to go to Chris. I still held on to a tiny possibility that this was all wrong, that I would get there and find it had all been a mistake, a dream, a scare. Anything but not real. Finally he asked whether I wanted to see Chris and I said yes.

I had to wear a sterile gown, footwear, gloves and a mask, as they feared I would infect him because of the state of his health. As I entered Room 10, and was met with what was left of what had been my handsome young husband, two things struck me quite vividly. First, that I did not have a husband anymore, he was dying, virtually dead. Second, I would have to be very strong for myself, for what was left of Chris, and for the girls. I didn't cry then. I moved towards his bed like a zombie. He was awake and recognised me instantly. He lifted his frail arm, the one which was not strapped with tape and monitor leads, and attempted a smile.

"What took you so long?" he asked.

In Hospital in England

As I write this I am having to fight hard to keep the tears back. I cannot understand how it was that I did not cry in front of Chris, then or ever. It was not that I did not have any more tears, for afterwards in my room I cried for a long time, until I fell into an exhausted sleep. I was grateful that the hospital staff left me on my own to deal with my sorrow. They kept a respectful distance, but they kept me under close surveillance.

The nurses were very afraid for me. I was impressed from the start by the attitude of the staff towards us. It was not long before I established that we were the only black couple on the ward, and their first heterosexual AIDS patients. Despite having two ingredients for stigma we were treated with such care and compassion that it left an everlasting mark on me. It was then that I resolved that if God would allow me time and life I would like to return some of this compassionate care to patients. Everybody went out of their way to be nice. Apart from the compassionate way they nursed Chris, bathed him, combed his hair, dressed his wounds, they each did small things for him, like bring him a flower from home, send him a post card when they were off duty for a few days, share their family photographs, and so on. I remember on his birthday, 23rd August, Sister Ann made a big cake with Happy Birthday Christopher on it. Everybody brought a card, and the staff came singing Happy Birthday. Although Chris wasn't happy at all, he managed a smile. This, his 36th birthday, was to be his last. I was so moved I went to my room and cried for ever.

There were times when Chris would be depressed and wouldn't talk to anyone the whole day. At first I would sit in the room and read to him, talk to him, or just be around for him to direct his anger against. Sometimes the nurses would take me away for shopping. Then I would feel better, buying small things for the girls, although I did not know when I would ever see them again.

In the second week the team was joined by the hospital chaplain, Father Storey, who turned out to be a great support for both of us. Chris loved him, and whenever he came around Chris would be cheerful the whole day. Father Storey would turn up with tropical fruit juice, and quite often he brought passion fruit. I don't know where he found them, so far from London. Even when Chris would be vomiting everything he took by mouth, when the passion fruit came he would eat them eagerly and did not vomit.

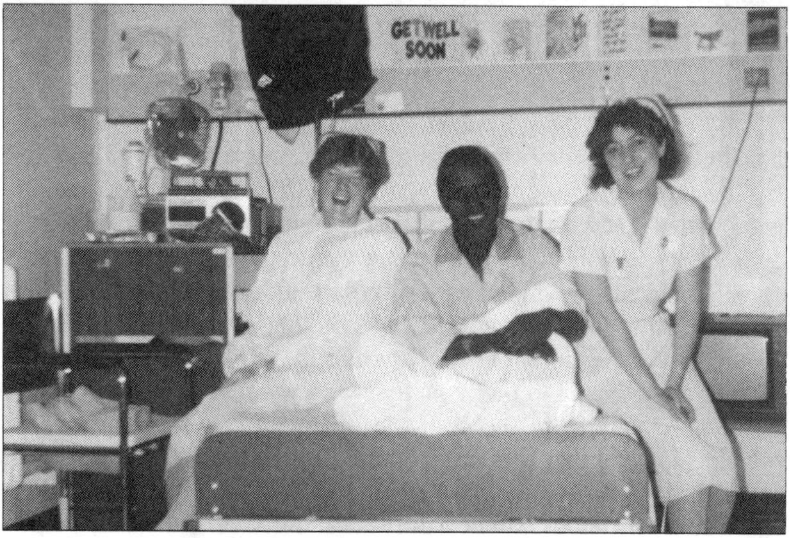

Chris with the nurses at Castle Hill Hospital

It was during the second week that Dr Nanda, the consultant, asked me if I would consider taking an HIV test. It was the first time that I realised that Chris being HIV positive had direct implications for me. Up to that time all that I had centred on was that he was dying. He was my husband and he was dying. I sat down with Dr Nanda and Dr Symonds, they explained that AIDS is a sexually transmitted disease and what the implications of this were for me. They asked me many questions, including whether I knew where Chris could have got the infection. I didn't. I couldn't think at the time. Then they asked me if Chris had ever had a blood transfusion. Yes. He had had a blood transfusion. Chris had been given eight units of blood when he was involved in an accident. He may have got the virus from that blood transfusion, which meant that he could have become infected in Uganda.

The Accident

I was at work on the 7th July 1983 when I was informed that Chris had been brought into casualty, bleeding profusely, having been run over by a bus. I rushed to casualty to find him on a trolley, his left leg twisted at a funny angle, and the doctor shouting for blood. In Uganda, like in many developing countries, blood for transfusions has to be found from relatives or volunteers, since there is never enough in the blood bank. I rushed around looking for blood donors. I was four months pregnant with Christine and unable to give blood myself. Two of my students agreed to give a unit each. I also rang all of Chris' family around Kampala and informed them of the accident and of our desperate need for blood. Godfrey, his younger brother, was teaching at a nearby secondary school and rushed in to donate a unit of blood. As he was the same blood group as Chris, his unit was transfused straight away. Chris had to be given eight units altogether.

Surgical repair of Chris' patella tendon and setting the leg in the proper position were followed by a long period of immobilisation in bed. I had to use all my skills as a physiotherapist to hasten the healing and subsequent mobilisation. This was my first real exposure to the value of true friends. My friend Mary supported me throughout this time, taking care of the children while I stayed in the hospital with Chris. In our country families often have to help patients with basic nursing care. He was hospitalised for two months and then discharged with a slight limp. Chris recovered slowly but surely, although looking back now I can see that he never really recovered his vitality. He was never the same man after the accident. It took a lot out of him. He seemed to just lose interest in life.

Later that year, in December, our fourth child, Christine, was born. I was working hard, and had an additional parttime job. Things between Chris and I had seemed much better since Marion was born, but by the end of 1984 we were having problems again. Looking back now, I know why he was feeling weak, but at the time I couldn't understand it. Chris seemed to have lost interest in work, and was frustrated by his lack of success in registering for a Masters degree. He had been making plans, before the accident, to go to England for further education. Often I would return home after my two jobs to find him in bed complaining that he was tired or not feeling well.

In November 1984 he developed a skin rash and sores in his throat. The sores cleared up, but the rash persisted for three months. A skin rash and sores were nothing to be suspicious of, so I did not suspect anything. Chris also seemed to have lost his libido, which I put down to his having lost interest in me. He was tired all the time, disinterested and moody. We were only having sex about once in two months. I thought he was afraid of having another baby, and, knowing how much he disliked condoms, I had an intrauterine device fitted. When I came home with the good news, which I hoped would excite him into action, he was really angry and it sparked off a big quarrel. During the early part of 1985 we seemed to quarrel more easily, and made up less and less. He also seemed to talk less and less to me, but found comfort in the children. I was frustrated and unhappy much of the time, and so the children turned even more to daddy.

This was when we started having major domestic problems again. In the time before he secured the scholarship to go the UK our marriage was in trouble. Essentially I thought he had another woman, and so we were quarrelling most of the time. At the time I couldn't understand why he was feeling so weak. Things were bad generally in Uganda at that time, and everybody was doing 101 things to make ends meet. This didn't help our relationship. I was working at two places, and I would only get home at about six in the evening. Chris would already be in bed. Those days he would go to the university, and then come home and go straight to bed. When he was asked why, he wouldn't be able to explain it. He would say "I'm not strong enough. I'm not feeling well. I'm not sick, but I'm not strong".

When the news came that he had been accepted at Hull University, we were all overjoyed. While he prepared for his departure we had a glimpse of the good old days. He was a happy, loving husband, and all the tiredness which had characterised the previous few months seemed to have just evaporated. We had a lot of friends, and we began to plan to build a house.

The news of the scholarship came at a time when Chris particularly needed it. His younger brother, Godfrey, had just died, in April 1985. Godfrey had been ill for about a year, from early 1984, with a skin rash, fever, loss of appetite, steady weight loss, and finally death from meningitis. Chris and Godfrey had been very good friends, so his death affected Chris greatly. We did not suspect though, at that time, that Godfrey had probably died of AIDS.

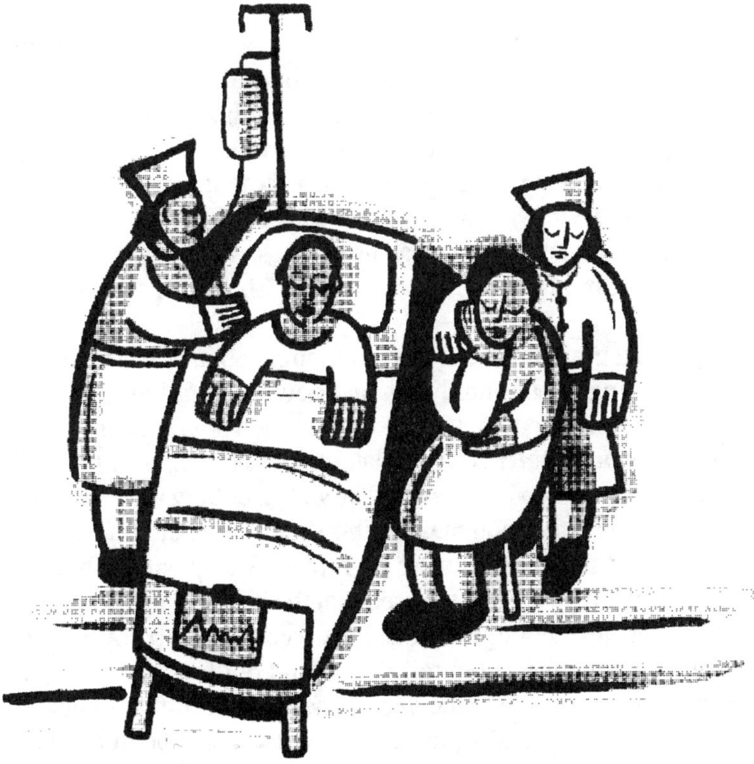

My HIV Test

When I was asked by Dr Symonds if I had had sex with Chris after the accident, and the blood transfusion, I couldn't tell him everything about the quarrels and irregular sex. There are some things you can't even tell a doctor. I told him that we had had a time of normal sexual relations after the accident, and he said that meant that I was at risk of being infected. I might also have the HIV virus. He didn't ask me if I wanted a test, but insisted that it was very important for me to know whether I was infected or not.

The next day a social worker was sent to talk to me. I don't know if she had been through a counselling course or not, but she rushed me through the whole counselling process - up to "What would you like to happen to your children if your test is positive?"

I was staying in the hospital at the time, in a bed just like a patient, in a room next to Chris. In the middle of the night I would look in to see him. Although there was twenty four hour nurse cover at his bedside, I also liked to check on him periodically. After they had taken my blood I started to feel anxious about it, especially looking at Chris and the way he was looking and feeling. That was the time when he started having very bad headaches. I cried a lot then, alone in my room, but I never cried in front of Chris.

I wasn't just thinking about Chris, I thought about the children a lot. I was thinking about him dying, and how I was going to cope with the children on my own. But after the blood was drawn I also had to think about myself. Six days later they told me, "I'm glad to say that the results of your test are negative". But they were very strict, very intent on not giving me false hope. From what I had told them they felt that the chances were high that I was positive, but that it didn't show up yet. They stressed that the results were preliminary, and another test would be needed six weeks later to confirm that I was in fact negative. I felt relief, but I did not feel happy about the result. In fact, the day I received the negative result it did not mean that much to me. It really didn't. I knew it was a good thing. I knew that from the nurses, everybody was so excited for me.

I didn't tell Chris about the result that day, and when I did tell him it was in a rather offhand manner. His first reaction was relief that I would be there for the children, although throughout his illness he was worried that I would marry again, or feared that I would become infected and die leaving the children with no one. He repeated this over and over. But from the day I told him the test result he started to plan for the future. The instructions were numerous. You have to do this. You have to take charge. You have to tell my mother this. You have to remember to tell my father that he should finish the house. You have to remember to do this and that.

Earlier Dr Symonds, the house officer, had explained to me the implications of Chris having AIDS, particularly the possibility that I might be infected myself. I tried to find out everything I could about the illness. Sister gave me what literature she could find. I spoke on the telephone to people in the Terrence Higgins Trust in London, and was put in contact with two people, Mark and Johnny, who were starting a buddy service in Hull. This was a kind of volunteer support system for people with AIDS. They came to see us and were very supportive and sympathetic listeners, although the issues that Chris and I were having to deal with were a little different from theirs as homosexuals. They spoke about the stigma associated with AIDS, but not having been exposed to it we did not understand what they were trying to tell us. Another source of support came from Chris' university friends and his professor, Bernard Jennings. Whenever they visited Chris he was very happy discussing the campus and their work. The professor encouraged him to continue his work as soon as he was better, and I believe that it was this feeling that he was needed at the university which encouraged him to make slow but steady progress.

Chris' major problem was still diarrhoea and an inability to eat anything. He was being fed intravenously. After intensive therapy with amphotericin B, the cryptococcus was finally cleared from his cerebral spinal fluid, and with intensive intravenous feeding with a specially formulated fluid he was able to restore some weight and enough strength to begin to get out of bed to be taken to the toilet.

Going Home

We were at the hospital for a long time, an agonising experience. Chris would get better, then he would be bleeding through the nose, the next day the diarrhoea would be less, the next week he would have a cough and fever. Through these ups and downs we received a lot of support from many different people. I can't even begin to thank them for what their support meant to us both.

But the time came when we started talking more seriously about the future. At first, I had understood that Chris was going to die. Then it seemed that, although his condition was too far gone for him to live totally normally, he would steadily recover and would be able to go back to university to finish his work. He knew that his only chance to complete his studies was to remain in England where he had access to medical care. What we totally underestimated was his need for support other than medical care. I mean the support that comes from family and friends.

We made the decision that I would go back home to the children. They were being looked after by my sister, and, although we were communicating with them regularly, their letters indicated that they were suffering from our absence. They weren't suffering materially. Chris' brothers, my sister, and Mary were doing all they could to provide for their needs. I remember when the time came for Elizabeth to have her first Holy Communion, Chris' brother Henry bought her a beautiful white dress and threw a big party for her. We saw the photographs of the ceremony. They were not uncared for. They were suffering because they missed us and because of the uncertainty.

I had taken photographs during our stay at the hospital, pictures of Chris at different stages. I put them in an album to send home so that the family could see what good progress he was making. What I didn't realise was that I had become used to his appearance. When the album reached home, and people compared how he looked in the pictures to the way he looked before he left for England, it only

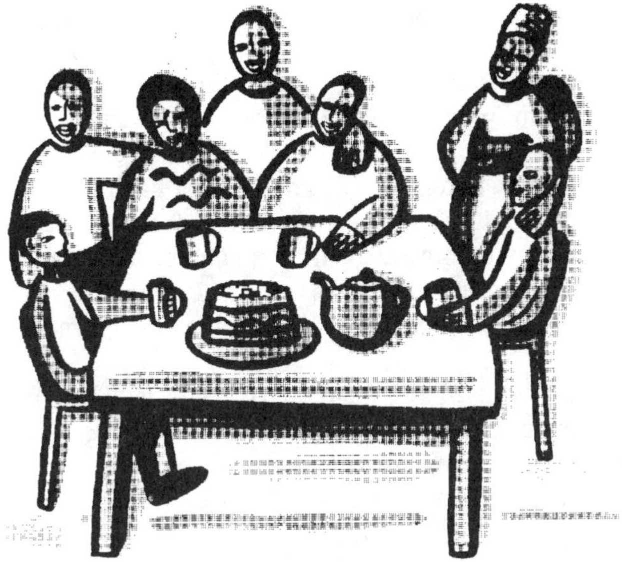

depressed them even further. By the time I got back everyone had lost hope and was convinced that he was dying.

My arrival home at the end of September was a very traumatic experience. I had left Chris in England knowing I might never see him alive again, and when I arrived at the airport I found a large group of friends waiting to meet me. I was very alarmed. I had not expected them. It was a working day and many of them should have been at work. There were my friends, including Mary and Florence, Christopher's brothers and sisters, my mother-in-law, and many others. They were wearing their traditional *Busuti* dresses and I wondered why they had had to do that. Of course my fear was that while I was travelling from Hull, and had been in the air overnight, Chris had died. What made it worse was that when I asked them why they were all there, they looked at each other and didn't reply. In our tradition, we do not talk openly about death. They didn't know how to give me the news at the airport. They told me they would tell me when we got home.

The airport is in Entebbe. We started to drive to Kampala, but branched off to my father-in-law's house which is halfway from the airport to Kampala. When we got to the house my mother-in-law, and everyone else, started crying. I was still afraid that Chris had died. I asked them again, and then they told me. My father had died.

He had died the day before. I was grateful that I had been in time, that I was able to see him before he was buried. But I was so hurt that he died just the day before I arrived back. I loved that man, he was very close to me, and I felt devastated. There were two very important men in my life and they were dying at the same time.

My father had been ill for nearly five years and had become wheelchair bound. I had been taking care of him. It was as if he felt that now I had another invalid on my hands I wouldn't have time for him. It was a big setback for me, and I was very lucky to have my family and Chris' family with me.

The urgency of having to support the children, having to work out the future, the urgency of getting on with life and preparing for the worst, may have helped me through the period after the death of my father. Also, the support and encouragement I received in England meant that I returned that much stronger and better prepared to face the world. Looking back now, though I was very hurt, I recovered quite fast from my father's death, because I was able to be at the funeral and I was able to give him a decent burial.

When I returned home to Uganda I found that things were not really the same. During the months I had been in England with Chris the AIDS issue had exploded in Uganda. Many cases were diagnosed but they were clothed in secrecy so that gossip about them thrived. People talked about them in moralistic and judgemental terms. Because AIDS is transmitted through sex, it was a popular belief that those infected must have been immoral and promiscuous. This was the time that I was first exposed to the stigma associated with AIDS and HIV.

The children started by telling me how they had been stigmatised at school, how people were asking questions about whether Chris or I had died of AIDS yet. I also began to notice that a few, not all, of my neighbours were very anxious to move on whenever we met them. Some of them stopped coming to the house. One or two neighbours tried hard to cover their anxiety and supported me in their own way. At the same time, I know that I too, in my resolve to stand with my head held high, did not make it easy for them.

I was beginning to feel the stigma myself. Whenever small or big things were done by others I felt it was being done deliberately. I expect everybody is exposed to stigma if they're in a situation like the one I was in. Some people don't understand, and you have to find explanations for the things that happen. So much of stigma comes from inside. People become so sensitive about everything that is said that even those who are being kind are misinterpreted as being nosey.

I went straight back to work and began to notice that some of my colleagues, too, were finding it hard to deal with me. I learnt that AIDS was being recognised in the hospital and was now being talked about. The Ministry of Health had plans to institute an AIDS Control programme, as an infectious disease. I had been prepared for some of the stigma by Mark and Johnny, my buddies from Hull, who told me the problems faced by gays with AIDS in the world outside Castle Hill Hospital. I had not been prepared for these reactions from my own people. I would walk into the staff room and people would suddenly stop chatting, suddenly it was time for everyone to get back to their work on the wards. I knew I was not included in conversations, or people would talk to me in very very excessively kind tones. I was surprised by this kind of behaviour from fellow health professionals who had access to knowledge and information, and who were trained to behave in a sympathetic manner. If they were unable to deal with me as an ordinary human being, how were they relating to their AIDS patients on the wards? I had to think back to my own training to examine the attitudes I myself had had.

My Work as a Physiotherapist

In my own career as a physiotherapist, in my work and interaction with my patients, one thing I am sure of is that I was a competent professional. I was given very comprehensive training by my beloved teachers, and my basic upbringing did not allow for a lack of discipline. What I do question now is my treatment of patients as people, as human beings with soul and emotions, not just as numbers treated and rehabilitated.

I remember working on the trauma and orthopaedic ward during one of the troubled times in Uganda. The whole ward was filled with young men in their twenties who had been shot and were wheelchair bound for life. Young men whose lives had just begun and had been stopped by a bullet. Suddenly they had no plans, no future.

I remember, vividly, that sometimes I would come to the ward with the best intentions, to teach someone to get out of bed into a wheelchair, to exercise his arms, expand the muscles of his trunk, so that he could cope with the chair. I would find him in a bad mood. No amount of coaxing or cracking jokes would get him out of bed that day. I would get very angry at this man who did not know what was good for him. I had a job to do. If he preferred to stay in bed for the rest of his life, he could suit himself. The following day, if he was in a better mood I would tease him about the tantrums. I had no perception of his feelings. I couldn't even begin to appreciate the various emotions he was going through.

At other times I would be part of a major ward round. Like teaching hospitals all over the world, these rounds included the consultant, registrars, houseofficers, interns, a fleet of nursing staff, medical students, nursing students, physiotherapists, occupational therapists, and so on. They would congregate around one case and the discussion would go something like this:

The consultant asks the registrar, "How is this man getting on?". The registrar looks at the notes made by the intern and houseofficers. He reports back. "Is he taking his drugs, Sister?" Sister consults the drug chart and reports back. "Is he in pain?" All these questions are asked and answered within the group. Explanations are shared by the group in medical jargon and no effort is made to include the subject of the discussion. Decisions are taken, and orders barked to the juniors: Take a chest X ray, change the plaster cast, begin partial weight bearing, give him matooke instead of pasta. Everytime someone says something the subject turns his head in that direction in the hope that he will be asked or will be given an explanation. In vain. Soon the whole group moves on to the next patient, and as it does so the subject may grab one of the friendly looking physiotherapy students in search of an explanation. All he may receive is a sympathetic smile, a shrug of shoulders, a promise to return later to answer questions. A promise which doesn't materialise. If he was lucky he may have received a greeting at the beginning which would have taken the form of "Good morning. How are you?" "Doctor how is this man?"

This kind of scenario was often described by Chris as the most inhuman part of interacting with people who were supposed to restore patients to full health.

Fighting in the Open

It became increasingly evident to me that if I was going to fight this disease in any way I would have to fight it in the open. Even Chris' own father had said that until people recognise and know that a person has died of AIDS they will continue to call it typhoid or something else.

I did not really have a timeframe or a definite plan, or know what strategies I was going to adopt, but the one thing that I was sure of was the decision to remain open. In any case I didn't really have a choice, because I had already told everyone, when I first received the telex, that Chris had AIDS. I suppose I could have retracted the information if I had really wanted to. I could have said that it was all a mistake, that Chris had cancer or tuberculosis. But I decided, quite instinctively, that I wanted to stick to the truth. It helped me that Chris and I had discussed it before I left Hull. I explained to him that I had already told people his diagnosis, and he felt it was the right thing to do. The crucial part was that he didn't feel that having AIDS was something to be ashamed of. He agreed it would be more helpful if we stuck to our original revelation.

I didn't go around continually telling everyone that Chris had AIDS. However, whenever I was asked what the prognosis was, that is whenever anyone gathered the courage to ask me directly, I was able to say that the prognosis was poor, that, because it was AIDS, it was only a matter of time before Chris would die.

I didn't really know what to do, but hoped for the best. I was getting information on Chris on a weekly basis, and he was making steady but slow progress. Just before the end of October 1986 I had another message from Hull, this time saying that Chris was coming home. Either he had been thrown out of England, which I didn't think was possible, or he had reached a state where he would not benefit from further treatment, which meant that he was coming home to die.

I was able to speak to Chris on the phone, and he told me that it was his decision to come home. I was surprised to hear that he was able

Why I came out in the open

I have been different, willing to share the experience of AIDS in my family, for a number of reasons. In the beginning I had already declared Chris's illness, and I couldn't retract that. I suppose I could have opted not to tell the world, just suffered in the family. But I was increasingly convinced that AIDS was a disease that shines in hush and thrives on secrecy. It was prospering because people were choosing not to talk about it. It was this realisation that provoked me to go wider, beyond my personal circle, beyond the people I worked with. The quieter we keep it the more people it will affect and stigmatise, especially while people believe that AIDS affects some people and not others.

I reasoned that if people could see how it affected us, an ordinary average family, not a poor one, not a rich one, just an ordinary normal young married couple, they would understand the importance of coming out. If it could happen to us, it could happen to anybody. The support that I received after Chris died was in response to my coming out. If I'd covered my head, been miserable and cried, I don't think I'd be where I am today. But also I wanted to talk about AIDS so that at least my children, and yours, would be spared. They would know and have information about AIDS before they became sexually active, and be able to talk about it. The price I had to pay for coming out, and it was a cost, was very small compared to what I would get by saving the children.

to eat, and the people at Castle Hill were going to give him the medication he needed to come home with. He wanted to be home and with the family, because he felt that without us life was just bare existence. In these circumstances I couldn't argue with him about the need to be near excellent medical care. We also badly wanted him to be home with us.

I was very excited at the prospect of his coming home, but I was also very apprehensive about how he would cope with the stigma I had already experienced. I was counting on his family, his brothers Henry and William and his sister Margaret, who were very supportive. When I told them he was coming home, they agreed it was for the best.

I can't describe the atmosphere at the house. The girls were so excited. We decided that we would do some major cleaning and fumigation, as the need for a clean, bacteria free environment for Chris had been stressed while I was in England. The girls and I started scrubbing. We cleaned the whole flat. Every cockroach, every possible source of infection in the house, had to go. I know now that this wasn't necessary because ordinary household hygienic practices are quite adequate for people with HIV, but at the time it made us feel more prepared. By the time he came home the house was as ready as it was ever going to be.

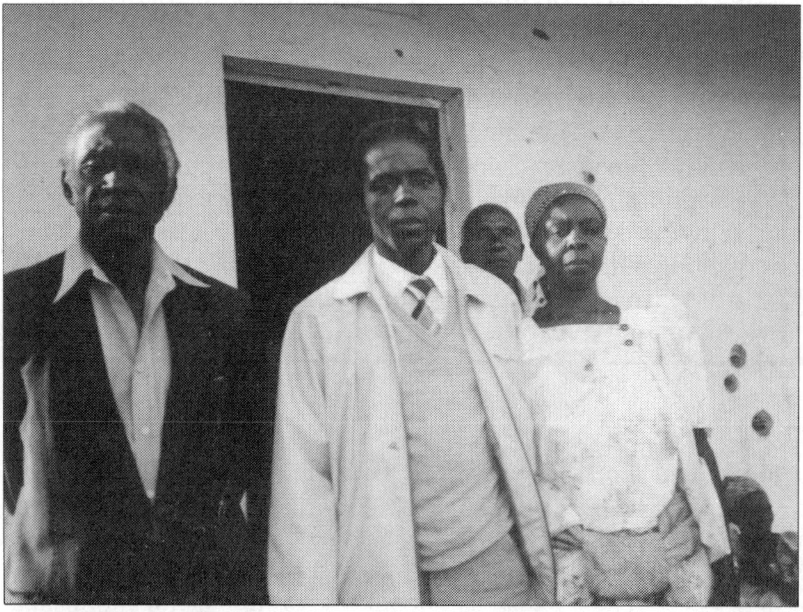

Chris' Return Home

The day came when Chris returned home, when he actually stepped off the plane, with the assistance of Jan Webster, a nurse from the British Council. I had arranged for an ambulance to be available on the tarmac to receive him, because I didn't imagine that he would come off the plane walking. When he did it was a tremendous boost, for me and for the whole family who were at the airport to meet him. We returned to his parents' house where a big meal had been organised. A big crowd turned up. The majority had come to sympathise, but there were some who had come to see what a person with AIDS actually looked like.

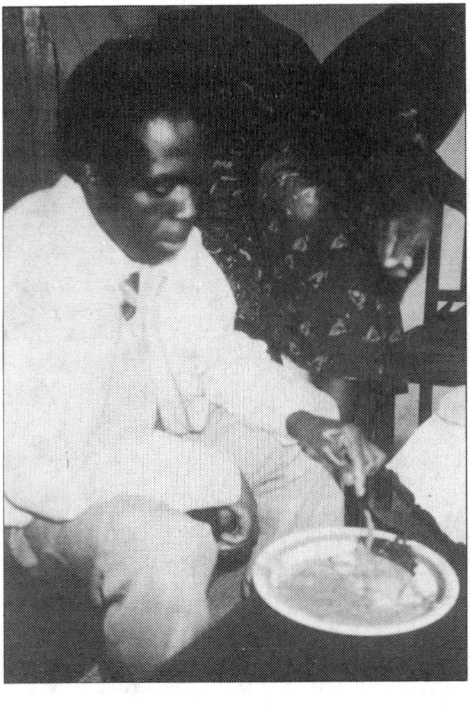

Chris handled the situation brilliantly. He was very excited, and he ate well. There is a photograph of him eating this whole mountain of food and he told me that the food had revived him. After this beginning he was able to eat small amounts of food, although he did vomit intermittently. That day the experience of seeing the children and his family gave him new life.

Before Chris came home I had held many discussions with God. I constantly asked him for a miracle, and on that day I feel He performed a miracle for me. Christopher coming home was like rising from the dead. From the hospital bed in Castle Hill to being able to come home was the first miracle that I can recall in the whole terrible experience. I was later to think that there was another miracle, my good health. But the first miracle was when Chris came home, and was able to live with us again, in our home. It was nearly two months before he became ill again.

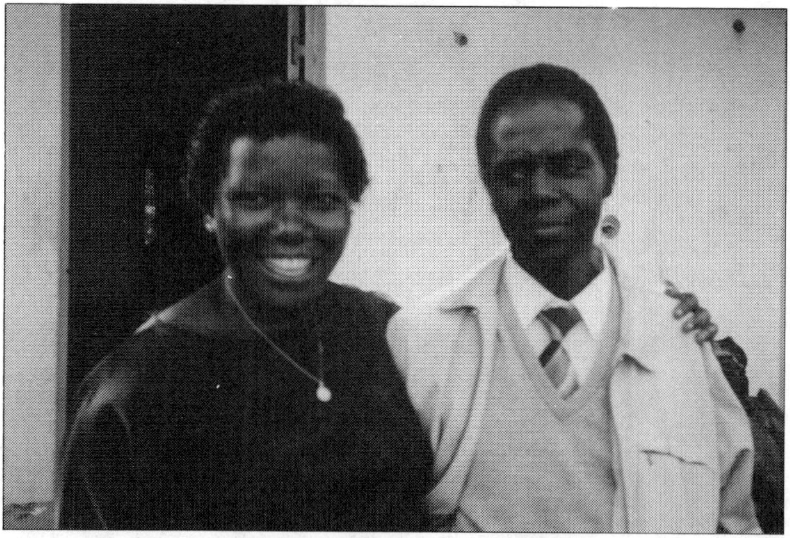

Noerine and Chris, October 1986

We had arranged that Chris would go straight to the hospital on his return. We expected him to be tired, and need time to recover his strength under medical supervision before he returned to the house. He was in hospital for only two days, but in that time we were exposed to what it was like to be known to have AIDS in a hospital in Uganda. Despite a private room with the best facilities Mulago Hospital had to offer, I was made aware from the outset of the extreme stigma that existed. Even the nurses were unwilling to come anywhere near him.

There were many people in the hospital who knew Chris from his days as a radiographer. There was a large influx of visitors, who mainly came to look at him, to see what someone with AIDS looked like. We had no privacy at all. There was another unpleasant aspect to these visitors. Chris was different from his ex-colleagues in that he had studied and worked hard to advance himself. Most of them had become stuck in their hospital jobs. Their attitude now was to gloat over his misfortune, after all he wasn't going to make it anyway. Even the doctor Chris had been referred to never came to see him. To the doctor there was no point in wasting time over someone who was dying anyway. Eventually an expatriate surgeon, Wilson Carswell, who was not involved professionally in his case, took over his care through kindness and compassion. I resolved then that, if he fell ill again, I would do everything possible to nurse him at home, rather than take him back to the hospital.

After two days he came home, and we were able to live a very close life as a family. It was as if we all knew that the time we had together was very short, so we shared our loads. Chris was physically very ill and a sexual relationship was completely out of the question. During this time I really loved Chris, but it was like a maternal love, a deep caring for him. As a family we were very close and loving. The girls enjoyed his company. Christine, the baby, always jumped into his bed and wanted to sleep with her daddy. Chris fixed things around the house. The whole month was as fruitful as could be.

I was prepared for a long, long period of illness, so I arranged to go back to work and organised things so that he had everything he would need within easy reach.

The Search for a Cure

On our return home from the hospital the struggle to keep Chris alive started. The whole family joined in, including Chris' family, my family and friends. A prominent feature of this time was the search for a local cure. Everyone started looking for herbal preparations that they had heard were effective. The biggest problems then were Chris' lack of appetite, vomiting when he ate solids, and intermittent diarrhoea. He was very thin and had a very itchy skin rash. However, the meningitis had cleared and he wasn't really in pain, which was a blessing. Chris was a very good patient and laughed and joked a lot with the children.

I had access to a pickup vehicle at the time. If I heard that there was a healer in a particular part of Uganda I would drive there and come back with a bottle or jerry can of preparation. I would go from place to place as people heard of effective healers and preparations. Relatives were bringing medicines by the jerry can too, and soon there were medicines for wrapping, medicines for sniffing, medicines for drinking at this hour, and so on. If anyone came to the house they would be struck by the long line of jerry cans of medicines, or the refrigerator filled with all kinds of bottles. Chris took all these remedies faithfully, alongside the medicines he had been given in Hull. We really hoped something would come out of all those herbal preparations.

Running from one place to the next in search of a cure, the one thing I never succumbed to was witchcraft. This was suggested many times. A traditional healer would be able to tell us precisely why Christopher had got this disease. The only reason I didn't go was because I am a Christian and so opposed to witchcraft. Otherwise, I can assure you, when you are dealing with AIDS you get to the point of desperation, in which even the most deeply felt principles are put to the test. If I had had any doubts, or if I had not been given the information and counselling I needed in England, I may have consulted a traditional healer. I knew Chris had an illness that could be explained scientifically, and it had already done enough damage.

I agreed to use the herbal medicines in the hope that they might help his symptoms.

It was during this time that we began to think about what we could do about AIDS generally. I started to seek out other people on the wards at Mulago Hospital who had been diagnosed with AIDS. When I met David he was actually nursing his wife, who died a few months later. I encouraged them to come to the house, just to talk or to share meals. I was away at work a lot and they became regular visitors for Chris. These were the meetings that eventually gave birth to TASO. Chris was the best informed person about the disease, having done a lot of reading on the subject in England. It was refreshing and supportive for the others to find a person with AIDS who had information and experience of the things that they were just beginning to go through.

This companionship provided some of the best times for Chris while he was at home. He felt that he could contribute to the wellbeing of his friends. When we talked about the future and setting up an organisation he was very receptive to the idea. He thought that he would be strong enought to start an office in town where he could receive people.

> I have been exposed to both sides of the coin of HIV infection and AIDS. I was exposed both to the extremes of kindness, compassion and care (as I had experienced in Hull), and to the extremes of stigma, lack of understanding, and rejection in Uganda, by the society in which I lived. It was this combination which prompted me, with a self support group of people with AIDS, to begin meeting, using our homes. My home was the first meeting place, even before Chris passed away. After he passed away we felt even more the need for a place for people with AIDS and HIV infection to meet, exchange ideas and share emotions.

Chris' Final Illness

Everyday, before going to work, I would make preparations for Chris, so that everything he required was within easy reach. He was a good patient, but at times he would get very bad spells of depression, and then it was difficult for us. He wouldn't talk for a whole day. Even though I had been prepared for the different moods that are likely to occur when someone is dealing with problems of this magnitude, it was a very difficult time.

I tried to deal with the problems as they came up. Sometimes Chris would react to his dependence on me by being irritable with me. Many women who are nursing their husbands experience this resentment, a natural and understandable emotion. We have to find the courage and patience to deal with it somehow. Chris would sometimes get possessive, not wanting me to go to work, but to remain with him to talk and to be a wife in the house. I recall this vividly because of the day he fell really ill again. I got up in the morning and, as usual, prepared all the things he would need in his room for the day. He was still in bed, but asked me not to go to work that day. I thought he was being belligerent, it was the way he said it. I told him I had to go to work. I hadn't warned the others that I wouldn't be coming, and my duties wouldn't be covered. He should have told me the day before if he didn't want me to go. He insisted that he didn't want me to go to work, and threw what I thought was a tantrum.

He asked how he could get better if he didn't have somebody constantly to look after him. I replied that we wouldn't have any money if I didn't go to work. It was a small domestic quarrel, but it showed the kind of communication failure that can happen when you are caught up in something. After I had arranged everything I went to work. Perhaps I didn't react with compassion that day. If I had stopped to ask him why he was feeling like that he may have told me that he had had a bad night and that he had a fever. I may have realised how insecure he was feeling. So I went to work and explained to my colleagues that Chris needed me that day.

When I came back at lunch time he was very ill. He was feverish, with a temperature of about 40 degrees, and had collapsed in the bathroom where he had gone to get a wet towel. We had a houseworker, but Chris knew she was afraid of him, afraid of the infection. My sister was also there, but he was stubborn and wanted to do things for himself. The only people he ever asked to do things for him were one of the children, Betty or Phiona, or me. Even then he worried about infecting the children. He knew intellectually that the virus was not spread through household contact, but he insisted on disposing of his dressings or vomit himself. He cleaned his toilet himself. He was very particular and fussy about these things. He also said that he didn't want to be a burden to others.

I helped him out of the bathroom, took him back to bed, and realised that he was very ill. I gave him some medication and went for a doctor, who said that he had pneumonia and started him on a course of antibiotics. The fever persisted for the next few days. I sent a message to his mother, who came immediately, with his sisters. He started vomiting and complaining of a headache. This was a persistent headache that didn't respond to pain killers. When he also started having diarrhoea we put up an intravenous drip. I was quite determined to nurse him at home, as far as possible. As a result of our earlier hospital experience I wasn't happy about the idea of taking him to a hospital. I nursed him for 10 days, but he didn't get any better, and eventually he started to cough up blood. We realised that he needed a blood transfusion, and there was increasing pressure from the family to take him to hospital.

On the tenth day, I can't remember the exact date, it was sometime in November, we went to the hospital and he was admitted and transfused with two units of blood, which seemed to revitalise him. His temperature subsided, but the cough and the diarrhoea didn't improve. He grew weaker and weaker. He was in hospital from that time until January 1987, getting worse and worse. On the 23rd January he died. He died in great pain. A week before meningitis had been confirmed again. He had relapsed. We had feared that happening all along, because we knew that the drugs he needed, the drugs that were effective against that kind of meningitis, were not available in Uganda. They were too expensive. I knew when I was told that there was a relapse in the meningitis that the end had come.

He was in great pain. I can't even begin to describe the kind of pain he was in. He had this terrible headache, which lasted for five days. He never lost consciousness. He suffered all that pain, and we felt the pain with him. The children would come into the room and he would ask for a wet towel to be put around his head. Even today my baby Christine, who was barely three at the time, remembers daddy's headache, and if any one says that they have a headache Christine becomes very anxious. If I have a headache I don't always tell her, because she has very bad memories of that headache.

Our experience with the hospital staff was an uncomfortable and distressing one. They did not know how to help us in a compassionate way and their personal fears and prejudices were predominant. The nurses would arrive as a team, on their routine ward rounds, and stand at the door to our room to greet us with their hands held behind their backs, not daring to cross the threshold. I became defensive and reluctant to ask them for anything, because of their manner.

Everything, all the nursing, cleaning, feeding, and caring, was done by my mother-in-law, Chris' sister, my friend Mary, the girls and myself. Even when the intravenous fluids needed replacing, or if the canulas needed resiting, it was up to me to find a doctor to attend to it. Often I would try to do it myself. Soon all the veins were too damaged to take the intravenous canulas. I persuaded the junior doctor to attempt a cutdown. This is a minor surgical procedure where the skin in the leg is cut and the vein exposed for direct introduction of the canula. The doctor was not experienced in this procedure which was rarely done, but Chris was very dehydrated and desperate for fluids. I scurried around to find the cutdown set in the hospital stores. The nurses who should have been assisting were standing at the door watching curiously. One of them made a comment I have never forgotten, "Imagine such a fuss being made about someone who is already nearly dead, a skeleton with AIDS".

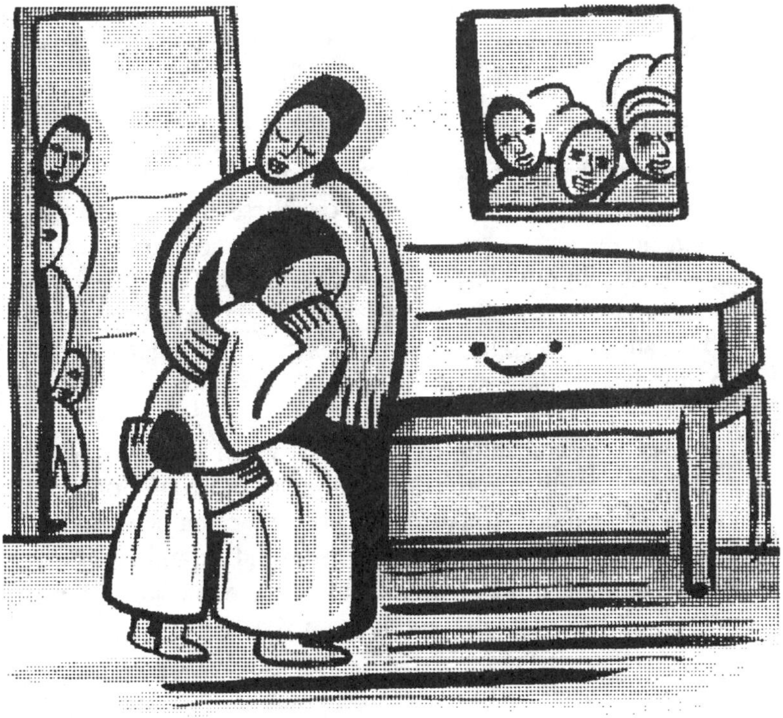

All this time Chris was awake and in agony, begging us not to hurt him anymore, promising he would do his best to drink and not vomit. The doctor and I did the cutdown, I was reading from a textbook and the doctor was following instructions. This provided Chris with the fluids he needed for 48 hours, which was when he died.

He died in a lot of pain, and this is something that I cannot take. Even today. I can't understand why he had so much pain. He had withstood so much, and he could have died peacefully, but he didn't. He died in a lot of pain. It was too much pain, and afterwards I couldn't take it any more. I couldn't take it. I was surrounded by family and had a lot of support, but after the funeral I went away. I was completely devastated. I had known all along that Chris was going to die, but I wasn't prepared for the way he died. Such undignified pain and suffering. So I went away, to my mother-in-law, away from the house. I wanted to be near the place where Chris was buried. I was away from home for three weeks.

> Sometimes, when I'm talking about these things, like the headache the week Chris died, I relive the moment, and the pain is deep in my bones. I have a feeling that my daughter Elizabeth also responds like this. She would just sit and look at her father, especially when he was in agony, when he was vomiting, when he was so ill.
>
> There is a special thing that happens when vomiting with AIDS. You begin to vomit, and just vomit and vomit forever, even if all the food is finished, you just keep retching. I would hold Chris and hold him, he would go on and on, and then start sweating, until he lay down exhausted. When I think about this, it still brings goose pimples to my skin.

TASO: The Beginning

Elizabeth, Phiona and Marion were at school so I gathered up courage and went back to work. I soon discovered that I couldn't function in the same way as before. I couldn't carry on working as if nothing had happened. I decided I had to concentrate on supporting people with AIDS who were going through the experience I had gone through. By this time some of the original people I had contacted had already died of AIDS.

After Chris' death and my return to work, I began to plan for the future. Despite having taken a test, and had a negative result, I did not believe that I was free of infection. I first asked God to give me a little more time. I specifically asked God to give me one more year, to see whether I could use that one year to do something useful for people with AIDS.

I managed to trace David, Jason and Jane, some of the people who had originally met with Chris, and made contact with others who were infected with AIDS. We started meeting again, and talking more constructively about starting a support group. At first we met at my house, Cheshire Homes, or in my office at the School of Physiotherapy. Initially the group was big, but it fluctuated, becoming bigger and then smaller, bigger and smaller, as members of the group died and new members joined it. Within the first group I was the healthiest. I decided it would not be useful to share the information about my test in England and the negative result with the others. Whenever I was asked, I said that I hadn't taken a test. This way the group could relate to me better than if they knew that I had had a negative result.

At first we met informally, sharing whatever information we had. Then we began to get information from organisations like the Terrence Higgins Trust in the United Kingdom. This went on until we began thinking seriously about starting an organisation. We didn't know then what we would do for money. We were not aware of the possibilities. However, as we reached out to other people who

I have chosen to conduct myself as if I am infected. Whether the results of an HIV test are positive or negative, we need to conduct ourselves in a way that either does not infect others or so as not to get infected from others. It is not the test results that are important. It's what we do with the results, how we conduct ourselves - to avoid infection or to spread infection.

Sometimes I think I should take another HIV test. If it came out negative it would reassure my children, but otherwise what difference would it make? Although I had a bloodtest which was negative, the fact that I have been exposed to infection makes me unwilling to take a second test.

After Chris died there was talk of my having AIDS. Would I die soon or not? More information was becoming generally available on AIDS. People were learning more about it. Everyone knew that if a man died of AIDS then his wife would die of AIDS soon after him. It was not a question of whether I would die, but when, as though everyone was waiting for me to die. I hadn't told people that I had had a test. I didn't think it would be useful, and I didn't think people would believe me. In any case, I had been told that I had to have a repeat test to confirm the first one.

I must say the test, even though it was negative, didn't mean much to me. I didn't believe the result. Initially I simply didn't understand what it meant, but later, having learnt a lot about HIV infection and AIDS, I couldn't believe that I could be genuinely negative. I chose to conduct myself as if I was infected. This is still the way I conduct myself today.

were infected, we found that a lot of the time they didn't have food, or medicines, or transport to the hospital. Helping to meet these needs began to stand out as an important aspect of starting an organisation.

We realised that we would have to obtain government clearance to start an AIDS organisation. In October 1987 I went to the Director of the AIDS Control Programme (ACP) in the Ministry of Health. I told him about my husband having died of AIDS, and of our intentions. He was skeptical about whether I really had the courage to carry the idea through, and went through the implications of starting an organisation, particularly where the money would come from. I said that as an NGO we would look for donations, but we already had a group of committed people. Much to my surprise, he told me to go ahead. He only asked us to go back and write it down, and he would give us the support we needed. One of our group, David, wrote the ideas down as a proposal, and we received the ACP endorsement. This was a tremendous boost to us because it gave us confidence in what we were doing.

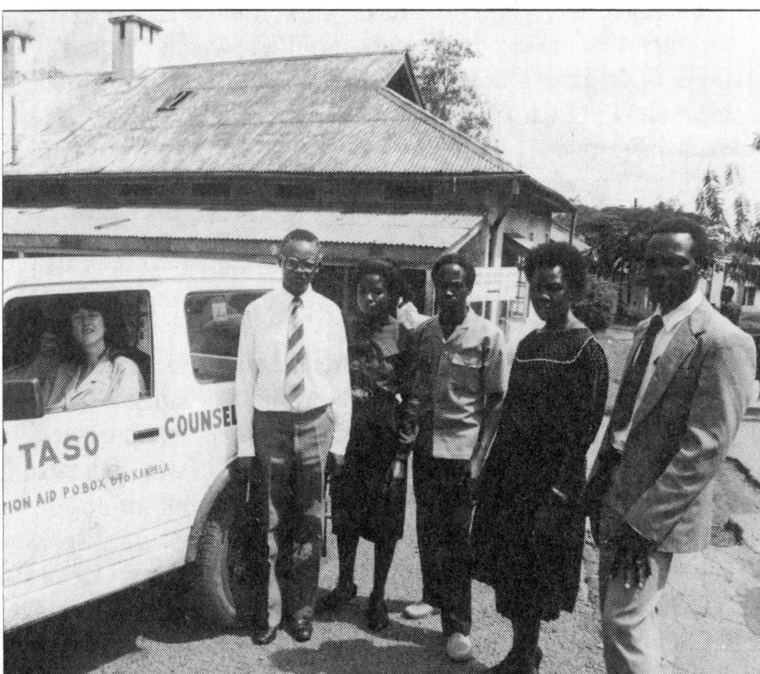

Early TASO volunteers

The Joy of Working in TASO

I have great respect for my friends with HIV and AIDS, who, despite being ill, in pain and suffering, being stigmatised and ostracised, worked with me to form TASO. I can recall that some of them suffered great pain towards the end of their lives, and it has been my continued sustenance to see other people with AIDS continue to become involved in the work of TASO.

One of the joys of working in TASO has been to see people come to us in pain and despair, and then see them happier and with hope after being offered counselling, even though they are still suffering physically.

Another joy has been the recognition of the potential for good in every person, good that can be tapped, stimulated, and encouraged. In TASO we have worked with people in the military over the last three years. Soldiers, whom we usually think of as having been trained to kill and so can be brutal, have shown great kindness and compassion to others. We even have one or two people working with us who were soldiers. They have seen and experienced the difference that kindness makes.

We were fortunate at this time, towards the end of October, to meet the Director of Action Aid in Uganda, Colin Williams. I had kept my friends in England informed about the group, and our need for funds to begin work. They introduced me to Colin who came to one of our meetings, just to listen. I think he was able to detect the infectious enthusiasm of the group, despite the fact that we were people with AIDS who didn't have a guaranteed future. He asked us to write a small budget proposal and gave us some small support to begin with, promising further support if we could demonstrate what we could do. With this assurance we started getting very involved.

David's wife had died, but he was working as an accountant and therefore was relatively well provided for. He had a car, and I had access to a pickup from Cheshire Homes, so we (David, Jason and myself) started using this transport to visit patients in their homes, bringing them to hospital, taking them home, mobilising people, etc. These demonstrations of kindness increasingly drew people to the small office we had loaned form Mulago Hospital. We all still had jobs, so we were generally in the office at weekends, and for part of the day during the week. We were later joined by doctors who started seeing patients with AIDs.

We realised the need to give people a professional counselling service, and sought and received sponsorship form Action AID for Dr Katabira and myself to go to the Centre for Advanced Counselling in London. This was my first training in counselling. At this course we were exposed to the basic principles of counselling, and to the ways of setting up an NGO.

We had formally founded the AIDS Support Organisation (TASO) in 1987 with 16 people, including 12 people with AIDS. One of the disturbing features of our start was that within one year all 12 of the founders who had AIDS had died. But in the same year we registered 850 other people who had used our services. In our experience and work with TASO we have found it necessary to maintain a balance of people with HIV and AIDS and those who have not been tested, to maintain a continuity in the services offered.

This was the beginning of TASO.

Today TASO is a fully fledged NGO, offering counselling services, outpatient clinical care, and homecare for people with AIDS and HIV infection. It also offers awareness and sensitisation programmes for a cross-section of the community, from medical personnel and political leaders to village community workers. We in TASO want to share with the world, especially our fellow Africans, our concept of counselling and support for people with AIDS, and support for communities that find themselves unsure of how to react to AIDS.

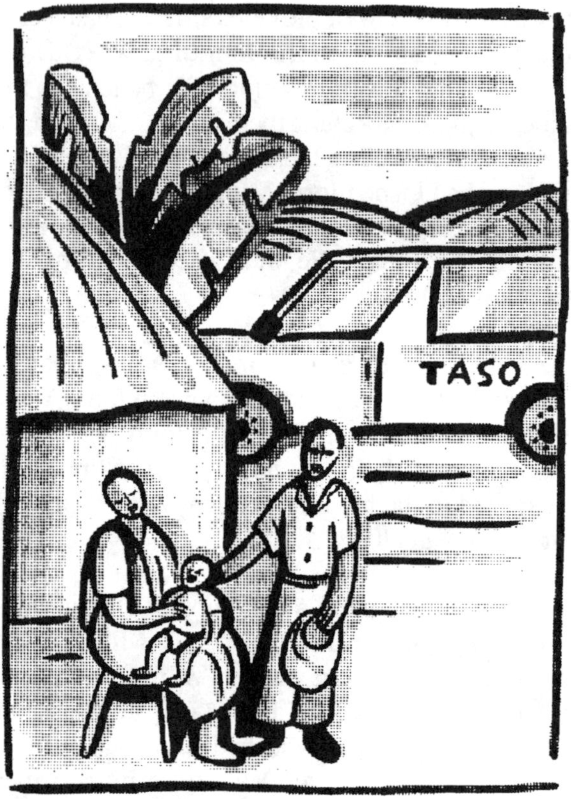

When we began we were just a group of lunatic people, some of whom had AIDS. We met to talk, to cry, to pray, to share, to let off steam. Soon we realised we needed to do more than that, especially in relation to medicine and clinical care, professional support, and welfare support.

AIDS and HIV infection thrive on stigma, on whispering and turning against people who find themselves HIV infected. By working together in TASO we have managed to prove to the world that it is possible to involve people with AIDS, people like me who have lost family to AIDS, and other people who have been personally touched, in campaigns against the disease.

AIDS took my man away and since then it has come back many times taking from my side young men and women, many of whom I have known and worked closely with as we developed TASO. I live with the agonising fears and the question of when, where and how might it come for me.

I have, however, opted to live positively with these fears, fight in the open, contribute as much, for as long as I can live, to the fight that will eventually lead to HIV's defeat. We are all called, therefore, to join in this war.

Keynote Address to the 2nd Workshop on Women and AIDS in Africa, Lagos, Nigeria, 28th-31st May 1990.

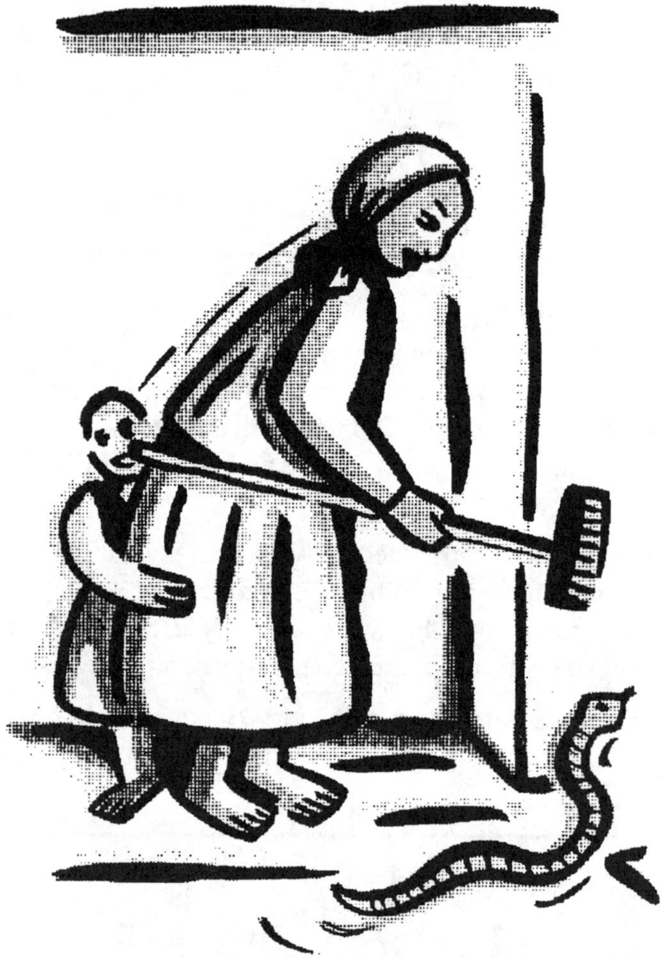

There is a saying in Uganda:
If a snake comes into your house do not waste time asking where the snake came from, but kill it first and ask questions afterwards.

Love Carefully

As we began TASO, AIDS was becoming recognised throughout the world. People were beginning to react, to begin initiatives to respond to the epidemic. A lot of these initiatives were geared to prevention. This was a good thing because, in the absence of a cure, prevention is the better way to fight this illness.

The public health messages that were being used then had a serious shortcoming. They all said don't catch AIDS, if you do you'll die. Messages like "Beware. Don't catch AIDS. AIDS KILLS". One popular slogan still used in AIDS control in Uganda is "Love Carefully", or the church slogan "Love Faithfully". The campaign based on this slogan contributed to the stigma associated with AIDS by relating it to low morals and death. By the very phrase "love carefully" is implied that the person who has AIDS has loved carelessly, even if this is not said directly. People who have caught AIDS have somehow deliberately gone out of their way to get AIDS, rather than avoid it.

These slogans were coming at people in Uganda left, right and centre, as part of a massive campaign begun in 1986. The messages were all the same. There was nothing for the person who was already positive and diagnosed with HIV infection. As a result of these early messages many people with HIV and AIDS reacted adversely. We in TASO had to really struggle to keep going, not only with the physical illness in our family but also with the mental torture and torment of these people.

Much as I appreciate that it may have been necessary to use messages that would shock people into realising the seriousness of the AIDS problem, this was done without realising that many people had already been caught. In this situation, with a love carefully campaign, when you meet someone with AIDS the reaction is to stigmatise them. To say, look these are the people who have loved carelessly. This may be particularly stigmatising in a society like Uganda which is almost 90% Christian. The Christian stress on moral values, even speaking against polygamy, can contribute to stigma in this situation. Although interestingly, when Uganda was, a year later, introduced to supplementary slogans with different messages, they came from a church hospital programme in Zambia, from Chikankata Hospital. These were slogans like "You can't catch Aids through casual contact", "Be compassionate to a person who has AIDS", "Be friends", that kind of thing. These slogans came a little too late, the original one had already taken root.

TASO began as an organisation which would provide counselling and support facilities for people with HIV infection, and preventive counselling for families and communities. It aimed at impressing upon people in the community, especially at the grassroots, that the person who has HIV infection or AIDS is not dangerous. They need our compassion, our concerted effort to be supportive. We need to be in a joint fight against the disease. The emphasis is on positive living.

Loving Faithfully. Where Does It Start?

With the advent of Christianity, and the education of women, some women are having more say in the house. They are not as accepting as they had to be in the past. In this changed situation one of the first things the woman says is "If I ever catch you with another woman, I'll kill you". The man really loves his wife, and he doesn't want to offend her. He knows that she is serious, and that she will kill him. At the same time polygamy hasn't left him, it's only suppressed by the circumstances and will remain so for as long as they are happy. Let me describe one possible scenario in this kind of relationship. Something happens at home, the husband and wife have a quarrel in the night and he wakes up and goes to the office in a bad mood. There, he finds someone of a lower status in the office who is nice and kind and is looking for a man. She is not looking for this particular man, but he sees this seemingly happier person. A relationship begins to develop, but one of the first things he says to the girl is "Look, I have a wife, and I don't want her to know about this relationship", and she accepts it.

Inevitably the girl is of a lower class, and values this access to the boss, so the relationship builds. He doesn't go to her often, he goes there when there is a quarrel in the house. Soon the girl feels very elevated. She has the boss, this highly educated person, and she might decide to have a child. The child remains in the background, the girl knows he has a wife, and agrees to remain in a secondary role, not make any noise, but she's not really happy, she also wants a man of her own.

So another relationship starts for her. She meets a man who sympathises with her because her boss treats her badly and only visits her when he feels like it. The new man says he would be available whenever she wants him. So he comes into the relationship, understanding that her boss visits her every Saturday. Every Saturday he makes himself scarce. She is a kept woman, and kept by more than one man. Then, perhaps, the new man has another contact somewhere, and so it goes on. This happens in the majority of marriages that I know. I know many big men in this situation, not with one but with two or three other women.

This man we are talking about is a busy man. Not only does he have a family and children to take care of, but he has a job, which sometimes takes him to Vienna or the US, or wherever. I was talking to a man in this kind of situation, with four women, his wife and three others. He was scared about AIDS. What could he do now? All these women have his children. He said to me, "But my situation is not so bad because I don't go to these women often". He was willing me to endorse his feeling that he was not at high risk because he didn't visit them often, only once a month. Most of the time he spent with his wife. But these were his children. He has a real dilemma. Isn't it too late? So, he said, "When you say 'love faithfully', where do I start?"

If we tell people who already have a number of stable partners to love faithfully, what will happen to the other women? Has the change come early enough? What are we giving the others who are not the ones to be loved faithfully? What are we putting in place of the man they have been depending on? We tell him, stick to one partner, but which partner? The one he married in Church? What are the criteria? Why should he choose this one? What are the ingredients that took him away from the first wife in the first place? We don't know. If we are saying stick to this one, are we saying that the attraction for the others is completely severed, and that he won't be attracted to another person?

These are the issues I discuss with women who come to TASO asking for an HIV test. When you ask them why they want a test, they say they suspect their husband is seeing other women. They say that if they are negative they will leave him. I ask them what they are planning to do. They may say they will look for another man who will be faithful to them. They need to think about the fact that they won't know whether any other man they become involved with is infected or not, even if he seems to be faithful to them.

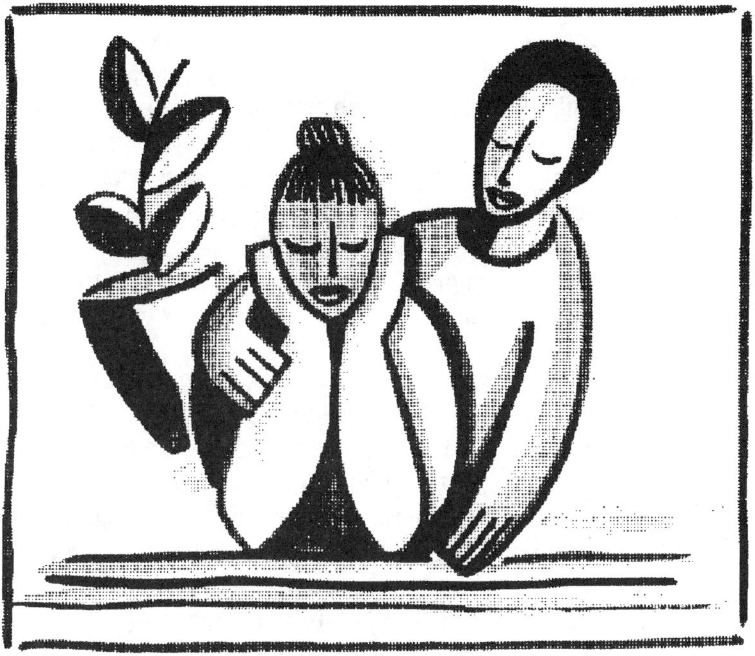

Polygamy is not conducive to the message of loving faithfully. When we say to a man who has five wives, love faithfully, love who faithfully? Another popular slogan is 'zero grazing', what does this say to a man with five wives? To make the situation more complicated, traditional practice has anyway become very confused because of Christianity, affluence, education, and so on. Wives used to respect each other and actually formed a very tight group. Today women, because of affluence, Christianity, or education, tell their husbands when they marry that they will not allow another woman in his life. When he finds one, the lies begin. This is the kind of situation that is bringing problems. The women will say they are happy to remain behind doors, but they aren't and so they look for somebody else who will not keep them behind doors, who will promise to be their own, and the chain continues.

Polygamy

There are many traditional practices that are in direct confrontation with the AIDS messages that we are giving. Culture and traditional practices are things that have been passed on from generation to generation, and we can't confront them directly by going to the people and saying "Stop, or you must perish". A better strategy is to educate them to realise that what they lose by releasing a traditional practice is much less than the risk they run of contacting HIV infection. This is a gradual process. A particular example in Uganda is male polygamy.

My father had eight wives at different times, and my mother married him, as his fourth wife, at the age of fourteen. She was given to my father after a wife had died in childbirth. She was so young that one of the other wives came to the main house to help her. She often says that she was actually brought up by her co-wife. My parents were married in the Catholic Church, although my father had kept all his other wives as traditional wives in separate compounds. My father was a chief, an affluent man, who always went to church. It was considered proper for him to have a Church wedded wife, but my mother was the only one he married in church. I grew up in a large family of four wives, two others had died before I was born and I never knew them.

I grew up, therefore, knowing and accepting the idea of male polygamy. Chris' father too had four wives (at the moment he has two). The idea of polygamy was not foreign to us, and Chris and I discussed it from time to time.

We had a very nice childhood by our standards, even though many of my brothers and sisters didn't stay at school long. My mother and two other wives stayed in the main house, the others all had their own homes. We each knew who our own mothers were, but we could go and sleep at each others house whenever we wanted to. I remember that as each of us came back from school, depending on who was nearest to you, you would eat your meal there and your mother wouldn't even worry whether you had eaten.

There were a total of 28 children in the family, including my father's adopted children. In my tribe there is a ritual where two men, if they loved each other, would cut their arms and then hold the cuts against each other to make them blood brothers. After this, if either of them died the other would adopt all his children and his wife. If in the ritual they said that all that is mine is yours, this agreement, for inheritance, would even supersede the claims of actual blood relatives. This was how some of my father's wives were inherited. When we grew up we were very careful never to discriminate between blood relatives and adopted relatives. I think this blood brother tradition has died down now, and I don't think anyone in my generation has practised it, but in my father's generation it was very common.

My father lived in the rural areas about 50 kms from Kampala. The houses of each wife were scattered within the same village location, not far from each other. My father had a motorcycle and he could easily move from one to the other, even in the same night if he wanted to. The interesting thing is that I never once saw him either going or coming from my mother's bedroom. They were so secretive, we could even imagine that we were heaven-sent since we never knew our parents to be in the same bedroom. I can't even imagine how he moved around, but he did because we were certainly his children.

In polygamous relationships it was assumed that women would not have their own sexual demands. If they did have affairs they were not talked about, so it's hard to know what happened. My father was quite old, about 50 years old when I was born, and my mother was much younger. Some of his wives would have been older, and would have stopped having children. Once a woman had passed her menopause, once she could no longer have babies, there wasn't considered to be any reason for her to continue being sexually active. This is very unfortunate if the woman is quite young when she has her menopause.

Teenage Sexuality

Before I met Chris, when I was about twenty years old and at the School of Physiotherapy, I had an affair with a man in his forties who was a friend of my older brother and my father. Right from the outset he told me he would marry me and, therefore, would protect me from pregnancy until I had finished at the School. I soon realised that my brother and father approved of this arrangement. Although I knew that he was already married, and in fact had two wives, the prospect did not alarm me. Being taken as a third wife, however, was not what I wanted out of life. So while I enjoyed his attentions and gifts, I was always looking for a younger man whom I could love and marry in church.

Even so I was infatuated by this man. If he hadn't been married I would have married him. I had just started my first year at the School of Physiotherapy and I was very flattered by his attentions. He would take his wife home at 5 o'clock, and then come back for me in his Benz. We would go out to eat, and he would buy me clothes and expensive presents. My only regret was that I couldn't show him off to my friends.

At boarding school, at about 18, the nuns had taught us that sex led to pregnancy, and that there were several different methods of contraception that could be used, including the condom. So when my friend suggested sex to me, it was in a very conducive atmosphere, I told him I was afraid of getting pregnant. He told me he would look after me, he would protect me because he was interested in my affairs and wanted me to finish at the School. I knew he wouldn't let me get pregnant because of his friendship with my brother and father. He had gone home to tell my father that he wanted to marry me. My father had agreed but said that I needed to finish my education first, because I was bright and needed a profession.

Although people say that men in Africa are not familiar with condoms, men of the world like my friend used condoms at that time, especially if they had families and were afraid of taking home an STD after going with prostitutes, or being troubled by young girls turning up on the doorstep with a baby. My friend also respected his wife too much to do that. He would never meet me openly, so we couldn't go dancing in case we met someone who knew them. We always went to drive-in cinemas or something like that. That's why I wanted to find my own man, my own marriage.

So many young girls fall into the trap of going out with older men who look after them, as I did. They end up either pregnant or with AIDS and thrown out of home. If one of my daughters told me that they were having an affair like mine, I would find the man and kill him! I asked my friend how he would react. He said he would kill the man who did with his daughter what he did with me! The situation is, of course, much worse now with AIDS. I do hope that my daughters don't get into a similar situation.

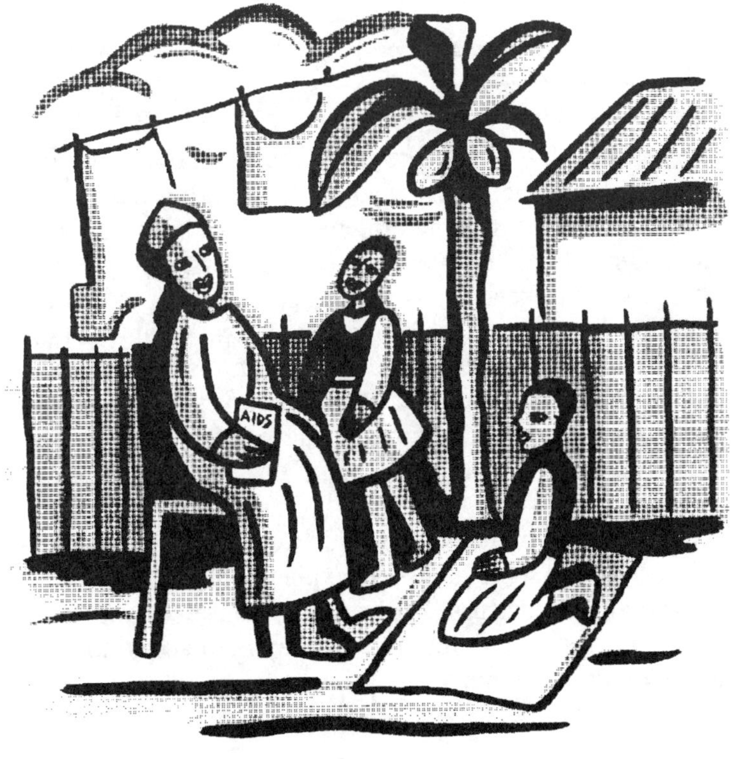

My early experience is probably why I feel that we need to give our children information. It is important to talk to them about sex. I never had any talks with my mother about sex. I had a talk with my paternal aunts, who traditionally give sex education to girls, but it was not very constructive - just that if you have sex you get pregnant, that's all. I think we need to explain to our children that sex is healthy, that the feelings they have about sex are normal, natural, and can be expressed without putting yourself at risk. They have to know exactly what the risks are. The most important risk is HIV infection, but second to that is unwanted pregnancy. I have tried to give the older girls the facts about sex and contraception, what protects against pregnancy and what protects against AIDS. I don't give advice, partly because of the counsellor instinct in me, but also because teenagers don't take advice easily. They listen and pick out what they need. What is important is that they receive straightforward, not distorted, information.

Some of the information we received from our elders was just lies. Stories to scare us away from sex. For example, if you sleep with a boy you wake up in the morning with a tree growing over your head, or if you sleep with a boy he damages you so badly that you smell forever - you get infected and go around smelling. That was my early understanding of sex, until I went to school and learnt better. So let us tell our children the truth, and then hope for the best. Mind you, I still don't think that I could hand a condom to my children. I would feel terrible morally if I did that, whatever age they were, and yet I know that it might save them.

Teenagers get a lot of their information from each other. Sometimes you go to tell them something, or to explain something, and you find they have already discussed it between themselves and know all about it. This is another reason why they need access to accurate information to pass around.

Talking About Sex

Women find it difficult to open a discussion of AIDS in the home. One option that we in TASO give women is to bring up the subject at an opportune moment, for example as they are sitting around the table after eating, not in the context of sex. At a first interview we provide people with pamphlets to take home with them. Using these pamphlets women can introduce the subject casually, "You know what, I was in the clinic and there's all this information about AIDS", and then begin to talk about AIDS. From this discussion condoms can be introduced, "It's said that condoms can also protect against HIV infection".

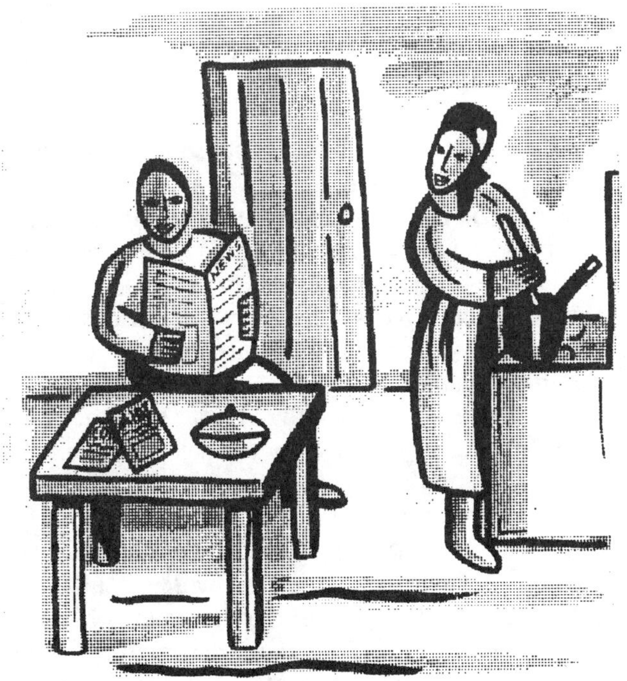

AIDS has brought two major taboos - death and sex - to the dining table.
Noerine Kaleeba, The Herald, 18th October 1990

Quite a few things not usually discussed can be raised, depending on how they are brought up. Recently I went back to the School of Physiotherapy to talk about AIDS. I asked the women how many of them had ever discussed AIDS with their husbands. Almost none had done so, and those who had tried to discuss it had done so in a negative way. They accused, “You, John, you really are moving around too much. You are going to bring AIDS into this house”. When you bring the subject up in that way you know it will lead to a quarrel. I suggested that they use the TASO pamphlet and introduce the subject as if they were just sharing their day’s experiences. Depending on how the husband responds, they could then ask, “Have you ever used a condom? The impression I got at the clinic was that these people were really serious about their campaign. They actually gave me condoms. Why don’t we try them? Let’s try them tonight and see what happens?” Bring it up as a joke, depending on the mood of your partner.

For some women, even through they are married, there’s no joking about sex. If there’s going to be sex, you will just jump into bed. In a situation like that you can’t just raise the subject. In my situation I could have introduced a condom. We didn’t use condoms often because Chris didn’t like them at all. But I think that if I had insisted he would have used them. We women know what tricks work with our partners. We know where their soft spots are. We know this, but we don’t use it to our advantage because we resent being the one to have to please him all the time. But with AIDS we have to, especially when we live in cultures where men control sex. In these cultures, even if you turn to your mother, and return to her beaten and swollen saying you won’t go back to your husband because you refuse to sleep with him, she will tell you to go home, to get out. How can you not have sex when he wants to have sex? A woman can’t win, and no legislation will change things until women have won men over to their side. Some things will be more acceptable if they are presented differently. We need to educate and sensitise people first.

Particular groups of women may have a particularly difficult task introducing condoms. Second and third wives, for instance, must try very hard to please their man when he only comes to them once a month. How can you present a condom in this situation, when he’s

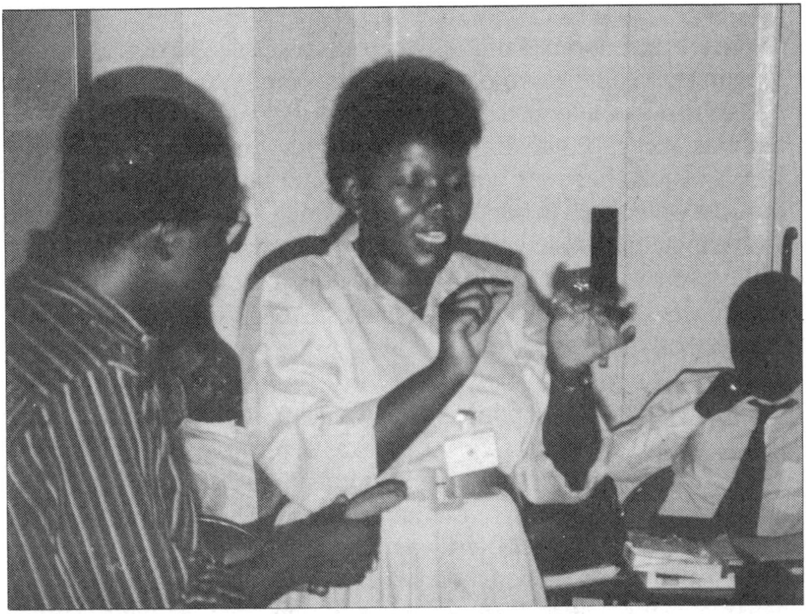

Noerine introducing condoms

visiting once a month? You can't. If the woman believes that this situation is right, she will not change no matter how long you talk with her. She will not speak up to a man, belittle him. She may believe that he should make the decisions. In fact, some women with AIDS say they have nothing to worry about because they got the virus from their husbands. Even though everybody in the village knows she is a faithful wife, she is happy and content that she got it from her husband. The fact that you have a fatal illness doesn't come into it. People tell me I am lucky, because even if I fell sick everybody would know where I got it from. The whole world knows that I got it from my husband. That's the judgmental part of it.

In my culture, once a woman is married to a man she has to have sex with him when he wants it. The only way a woman can remain married and in the same house is if she has sex when he wants it and the way he wants it. She can't negotiate for safer sex. She can't say that she feels frightened, unsure about him, or ask him to use a condom. The moment she asks that, he turns on her thinking that she has been up to something. A woman doesn't dare bring up the subject.

There are exceptional families where safer sex can be discussed and remain between the two of them, but, generally, if the man has not agreed to use condoms they can't discuss the matter further. In these circumstances, if the woman decides to stay in the compound, she would have to have sex with her husband or be thrown out. Even if the case were taken to her parents they would ask how she could live with a man and not have sex with him. It is out of the question not to have sex with your husband. So the only real choice for a woman, if she feels strongly about it, is to pack her bags and go. Where she goes nobody knows.

What are a woman's options if she wants to look for another man? If she's okay, ie not positive, the first answer in many cases is I don't want any other man, I don't want another man ever, or anything to do with a man. So in a counselling situation where the women has come in to request an HIV test we sit down and go through this. How sure is she? Even if she ignores her own sexual needs, what about her financial situation? How many children does she have? What would happen to them if she left her husband? Would he keep the children, take responsibility for them? Sometimes he would turn out both the wife and the children.

Usually it turns out that the woman is planning to leave her husband because she wants to find a more faithful man. In an environment like Uganda you have to ask whether she has ever actually seen such a man. Generally they haven't. They are just fantasising. Even when they see their neighbour walking hand in hand with his wife, they are just hoping that he doesn't go around with other women. Counsellors are trained not to give advice, rather to guide a client to work through the different facets of their problem. In this counselling situation, a counsellor will send the woman away to think further about the decision. If there is no other reason for the woman wanting a bloodtest, then she should think about whether she really wants to be tested. Many such women will decide, after thinking about it hard, that they don't really want a bloodtest.

In our culture there seems to be an assumption that women only have sex for babies or to please men. For example, it seems to be taken for granted that once women reach menopause, and can no longer

> In fact, in counselling partners who are negative when the spouse has tested positive I have yet to find someone who feels happy about this difference. For many people in this situation it means more problems, including guilt at being alright when he's suffering, when he's ill and in pain. You feel that you should be sharing the pain.

have babies, they don't need sex. I don't think women are only having sex for babies or to please men. Sex is a natural human desire, and has nothing to do with babies. For me the desire for sex is really associated with circumstances. When Chris was in England I knew that he would come back. If I wanted to have sex I would close my eyes and think of the day when he would come back, and how it would be. After he fell sick and I knew I wasn't going to have sex, I thought less about it. Psychologically I don't lie down and fantasise about sex, I don't have anybody to fantasise about, but I do get the desires, though not so urgently. Also I don't carry the process through, because my mind comes back to AIDS. Now I associate sex with AIDS.

A person with AIDS also has the right to have sex. Sexual relations with a person with AIDS, or HIV infection, is a matter for counselling. If clients with HIV come to me saying that they would like to have sex my first response is that it's their right. But as a counsellor, if a third person is brought into it, the partner, I would sit down with them and ask a number of questions: Are they infected? Are they uninfected? Do they know that their partner has HIV infection? What will be the eventual outcome? If the person with HIV infection is female, are they planning on having babies? They have a right to have a baby. It's their decision, but they need information and support to make an informed decision. I explain what we know scientifically about the risks, about transmission of infection from the mother to the baby, what it is like to have a child sick with AIDS. If she still wants to take the chance of having a child it is her decision and not up to me to talk her out of it. She will make up her own mind anyway and I want her to feel we are there to support her, not to condemn her.

STDs and AIDS

The stigma attached to AIDS is associated both with it being sexually transmitted and fatal, ie leading to death. But AIDS has been treated quite differently in terms of stigma from other STDs. It is now being reported that STDs in Uganda are going down. Fewer people seem to be going to clinics or private doctors for STD treatment. This is a good thing, as STDs seem to have a lot to do with HIV transmission in Africa.

The sexually transmitted issue leads to a great deal of stigma now, although historically STDs have been common in Uganda and not stigmatised, especially after the Second World War. At that time many people returned with syphilis and gonorrhoea, and made a point of bragging about it. They were not stigmatised. In fact there was a time among the Buganda, the biggest tribal group in Uganda, when the king caught syphilis and gonorrhoea, and it became a point of pride if a man had syphilis. In a group of men telling stories about how much exposure they had, you were less of a man if you had no story to share. While these STDs could be cured people could afford to brag about them. They only had to go to the clinic and get a shot. Even then, this boasting applied only to men. STDs were very shameful for women. Men brag about STDs, but who were they supposed to have got them from, who would they give them to? This example highlights the position of women in Uganda, even in Africa as a whole. Even today men turn up at STD clinics more quickly for treatment than women, who will suffer for a long time before they gather courage to come to an STD or gynaecology clinic. This has a big bearing on HIV infection, men come forward but women don't.

Promiscuity in Uganda is only understood in the context of women. A man can be promiscuous without being labelled as such. A man with multiple sexual partners is just a strong man, but a woman with multiple partners is promiscuous. The issues around STDs are the same issues around HIV transmission. Today it is not a question of promiscuity, it's just a question of sex. The level of infection in Uganda is such that every time you have unprotected sexual intercourse you are exposing yourself. Certainly most clients I have talked to have said nothing to make me suspect that they even know what promiscuity means. They have just been ordinary people who have had a sexual encounter which happened to be with a person who was infected, and they have become infected.

Prostitution in Uganda is not easily identified, because it is illegal and people will not identify themselves or others. Quite a few people sell sex for money, but many of them are also engaged in other activities. Some women set themselves up in a small house in a slum area and sell local brew and sex. I worked with two sex workers when we first started TASO, but not recently. But even then they could not admit, even in counselling, that they were sex workers. These two are the only two women I have met who sold sex for a living.

Inheritance

When Chris was in England we decided to build a house. When he had been away for about six months he started sending money home from his savings, and I began buying cement for the house. By the time he died the house was just being built. Today it stands exactly where he left it. It was an extremely ambitious plan, each girl would have her own room. Unfortunately, because of the inheritance laws in Uganda, and because I didn't have a son, my brother-in-law has inherited the whole property. Chris did leave a will, but it did not say much. As is the tradition, he left all matters to do with the children and me in the hands of his brothers and fathers. He didn't say "Noerine, you take care of the children". He said, "William, you take care of my family". In my tribe I am not expected to marry my husband's brother, but the family will expect me to remain a widow, and for William to buy food, clothing, and other things, for us. He probably wouldn't be able do that. He's been very nice, but he has a family of his own to look after, and is already struggling to make ends meet. However well intentioned he is, it is impossible for him to provide for us as well. Anyway, he is a lecturer, and what he earns is no different from what I earn.

At the time Chris died, and the funeral rites were taking place, I didn't think about the property, didn't even protest. Now I feel very badly about it. I have talked to my father-in-law, because Chris was building that house for me and the children. He was reluctant to intervene. This is our tradition. My brother-in-law has sons, and one of them will inherit the house.

I have begun to build my own house. If I fell ill today, if something happened to me, the girls would lose their father's house, just because they are girls. The moment I die it would be taken away from them. The first thing I did was to write my house into my will in the name of the girls. This way they will own it right from the start. If I don't leave a will the house I build would also go to my husband's brother, not even to my family. The minute a woman marries her family ceases to exist. One thing that this experience has taught me is that you have to fend for yourself. You have to put down word for word what you want to happen. This is not only my experience. I have seen other women less privileged than me who have been thrown out of their houses, every item (even clothing) taken from them, even things they bought for themselves, because they didn't write down what they owned, and what they jointly owned with the man. Chris knew that his family wouldn't take household property. They didn't take chairs and beds and tables. They didn't even take his clothes, they are still in his room. In fact, the girls wear them sometimes.

So, when I'm talking to people with AIDS I tell them to write down their things, write down what they want to happen when they die. It doesn't necessarily mean that they are going to die the next day. But many people are reluctant to write a will. They believe that traditional law is clear on inheritance procedures, and they don't want to create unnecessary conflict in the family. Unfortunately this solution may simply mean that the family conflict takes place after the person has already died, when the immediate family are left in an insecure position.

Women are beginning to get angry about these inheritance laws. Various laws are now being formulated to try to rectify them, and to protect women in their own right, for example we are strengthening the law against sugar daddies. But passing laws is not enough. There is need to empower women to recognise these laws, and use them to defend themselves. I mean, how does the sugar daddy law protect a girl who knows that the only way she can get nice clothes, and whatever else, is by going with a sugar daddy. She doesn't really have a choice, and she won't tell anyone that she is going with a sugar daddy. So the law doesn't protect her at all. It's more important to empower girls than to enact laws. It's the same thing with the law against rape. How many people get raped? How many actually come out and say I've been raped? It's partly because rape has a stigma. I'm sure many married women who get raped couldn't go to their husbands. The man, instead of sympathising with the woman, might take it very badly, and personally.

Fighting in the Closet

I appreciate the feeling that people with HIV don't want to be exposed, but how can we fight this infection in the closet? We can't. People are very happy to come to TASO and receive counselling and fellowship at the Day Centre, but if you ask them to come to a conference they say "Yes, I would like to come, as long as I don't have to speak like you do". In Uganda the only person who has spoken on TV and radio about being HIV positive, other than me, has been the musician and singer Philly Lutaaya.

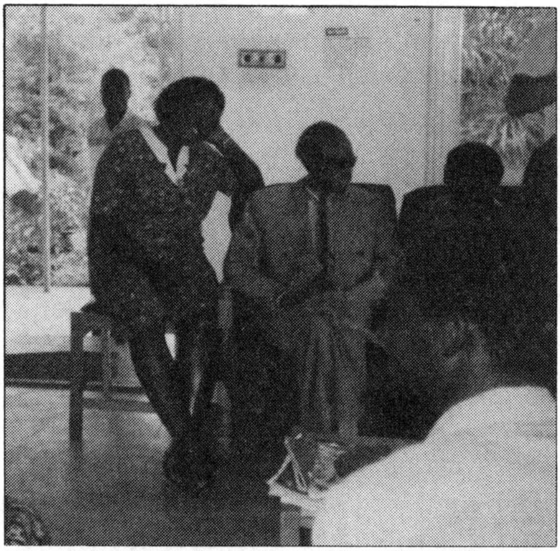

Philly Lutaaya meets members of TASO

Philly Lutaaya
Youth worldwide are a very sensitive group to deal with. We need messages that will reach them, and I think visual facilities are very useful. A video, "Born in Africa", was made about Philly Lutaaya, a very popular Ugandan singer liked by everyone. Once a man like that stood up and said "Look, I have AIDS", as he has done in the film, it had a tremendous impact on youth in Uganda. Not that every youth is now converted.

However, because our workshops in TASO are closed, people will come and speak to the people who are training, as part of their training. They seem able, quite easily, to discuss their lives in this situation. But it's a problem to get people to speak out in public, and I don't think that it's really the stigma for some of them. Some TASO clients have nothing from anybody other than TASO, ie TASO rents them a room, gives them food and a job. TASO is the employer, and the next of kin and relatives, as they would have been thrown out by their real relatives. Yet even these people are reluctant to do TV interviews. They will say "No. I don't want my parents, my people, to know". Yet, they have already been thrown out by their people, who already know about them. In Uganda people try to deny that anybody in the street can diagnose AIDS, especially full blown AIDS - but they can see it. Many people with AIDS cling to the feeling that AIDS is still confidential, or that they are still invisible.

This is a terrible thing. You know that people know, even though they are not telling you. You know they will continue to whisper about you as long as you remain closed. The moment you come out the mystery is broken. We have all seen the effect of interrupting someone who is talking about us. When you turn around and say "Are you talking about me? I see you are talking about this hump that I have on my back", you rob them of the joy of discussing the issue behind your back. They won't talk about you then. I explain to people with AIDS that once you are open you take a major anxiety out of your system. The perpetual anxiety of wondering who is talking about you, who is getting to know you have the infection, whether people know, what they are saying, is very debilitating. Fortunately I didn't have that particular problem because I had told people before I realised what I was letting myself in for, before I even returned from England.

Once I had returned, I could have retracted the news. I could have said it was a mistake. As a counsellor I see this happen every day. Sometimes, when counselling a husband or wife, I ask how the spouse has been, how they are coping. They say they will be better soon, the treatment is working. When I ask "Do you suspect that they may be HIV infected?", they ask "Is that what you think? Is that what you say?" Each of these people, I am 100% sure, knows their partner is HIV positive. I wish it was possible to impress upon people the need to make a commitment in the fight against AIDS, the need to give AIDS a face.

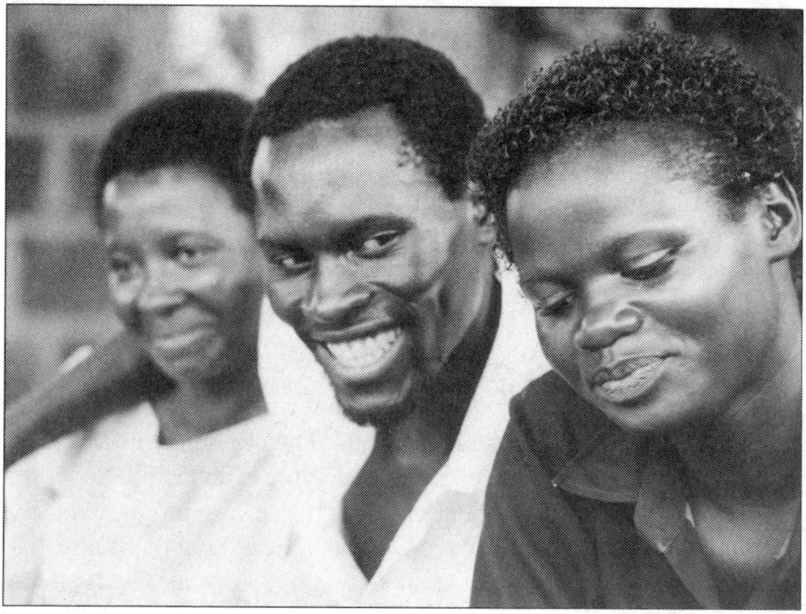

One way to deal with HIV stigma is to relate it to other stigmas, like racism or disability. I related the stigma to my own experience with the disabled in the Cheshire Homes. My exposure to, and my interaction with, those young men and women who were disabled, wheelchair bound or whatever, seeing how they coped, how they stood up to stigma, and how they really had to work hard to do it, was important for me in working with people with HIV and AIDS.

One of those young men was George Makombe. He was paralysed when he was young, from polio. He lived in a wheelchair, but he did O levels, A levels, and a university degree. When I was feeling very sorry for myself, after Chris had died, George came to the house and said "Noerine, I think you better fight it. You have two legs. You have two arms. You have brains. You have children. I don't have children at all. Every morning I go to work, I'm still paralysed, I'm still incontinent". He really gave me a shake up. After we had talked for a long time, I looked at my own situation again. Looking at George's experience and determination helped me to force my own determination to do something about AIDS.

It is very useful to relate HIV to dealing with other kinds of stigma. It even has implications for the way we have developed TASO. George worked with TASO as a volunteer. He has been trained in counselling, as an 'anon' (the 'anonymous' is our word for those who have not been tested, they may or may not be HIV positive). He was not, however, a fulltime counsellor because he had a job as a trainee accountant. On Sundays he would visit people with AIDS, especially those that were lying in bed feeling sorry for themselves. This is his special asset. He wheels himself in and says "I've come to see you. Are you getting up? Do you know that I've been paralysed for this long. I live in a Cheshire Home. I have a family but they wouldn't take me in." That kind of thing.

When you are dealing with the AIDS stigma you don't think there are any other kinds of stigma. This is especially so because the AIDS stigma comes a lot from the inside. You are so conscious of your status that even people who are just being kind are misinterpreted as nosey. But stigma does exist. It's all pointing fingers. Even though in Africa we may not have the discriminatory laws that some countries have, people are discriminated against. People have had their property thrown out of their houses because they have been discovered to be HIV positive. This has happened in Uganda, in the city. It's not that people are physically thrown out, but the landlord gets to know that you are infected and the next thing he does is try to get the house back. The infected people may say they can still pay the rent, but the landlords insist that they don't want the rent, they want the house.

Coming Out and Denial

> People take it for granted that I am constantly in a good mood, that I constantly want to talk about AIDS. Even if I stop at the petrol station to fill up they say: Now, what is AIDS? What is the latest about AIDS? What have you got for us? Where are the medicines? That kind of thing. Well, it's not true. There are days when I just don't want to talk about it. There are times when I feel that it's so unfair. Sometimes when I look at people who haven't been affected, or go to Church and see couples coming in with their families, mother, father and children, I feel so angry, so cheated, and I must ask, "Why me God?"

We try to protect our privacy by not coming out, and by not declaring our HIV status. This is one way. Our status is not written on our foreheads. However, there is a need to balance the advantage of privacy against the disadvantage of the anxiety of others finding out. Some high ranking people have even succumbed to blackmail from people who know of their HIV status. Yet they are dealing with an infection that can't be quiet for ever. When it flares up, there will be nothing that they can do to stop it.

The mind plays a very big part in how we deal with an infection like HIV. I know, if I am HIV infected, that one of the things that probably keeps me from having symptoms is the fact that I have brought AIDS out in the open. Yes, I do live in perpetual fear that I may become ill with AIDS. What I fear most are the early manifestations of HIV infection, particularly acute herpes zoster and meningitis because they are such painful conditions. I live in fear of that terrible pain that Chris had. I move around with a course of acyclovir (zovirax), a very expensive antiviral drug used for herpes infections, wherever I go, especially if I'm going away from home for a bit. I fear the infection and pain. I have to have it with me so the moment that I see a rash I can use it straight away. We keep a stock of it in TASO all the time. People use it as soon as they get a rash. If you start immediately it dries up the rash within two days, and it stops the rash from getting infected. However, we never have enough because it's very expensive. In fact, it takes up so much of our budget that we don't use it for anything but genital herpes.

Even though we fear AIDS like this I think that we do need to come out into the open with it. A lot of people could come out without too many repercussions. Seriously speaking, what could the repercussions be? It could mean getting thrown out of a job, or losing friends - but with full blown AIDS, depending on what firm they have been working for, they will have already lost their jobs. They already need help for basic needs. People will already be talking about them.

I feel strongly about the rights of people with AIDS, but we must accompany this with responsibilities. If it is my right to keep my job, it is also my responsibility that my job is done properly. Employers are being sensitised more and more to allowing people with HIV and AIDS to remain at their job, but the ongoing debate is the issue of productivity and production. It's all right if somebody is doing a job that can be done by someone else if they are not there, but production managers have factory quotas and targets to meet which cannot be met if some people on the production line are off sick a lot of the time. These issues have to be balanced up.

I remember counselling a friend who had recently been diagnosed as having AIDS. She was a policewoman, and had been working far from home. She was already ill, not just HIV positive, so living so far away from home and working as a policewoman wouldn't enhance positive living. I suggested to her that she seek compassionate leave, and think about moving, even coming to work with TASO. TASO is our organisation, it would be family for her. She insisted that she didn't look that bad, that people at her work place would not know that she had HIV. These people from work were the ones who had actually brought her from her station back to her home, and she was saying that they didn't know. I found myself becoming a little impatient with her, more so because I didn't have much time to sit with her. It's very hard for a person in my position to understand this behaviour. I get so frustrated, but I do understand. This lack of openness is a big stumbling block to the fight against AIDS.

We can't fight AIDS in the closet.

The Children

My children are comfortable around people with AIDS, and were from an early stage. They recognised AIDS as an illness. They know that AIDS carries a stigma, but for them a person with AIDS is just another person. My work with disabled people at the Cheshire Homes had already given the children a kind of empathetic background. I would often take the children to work with me over the weekend, and they would sit and read to people who were paralysed and bedbound or in wheelchairs. So they were prepared in a way for the work I do today. I don't hesitate to invite people with AIDS to the house, and the children don't make them feel any different to other people. Christine, the baby, will be the first one to jump into their laps. So I know it was a good experience for them, although in many ways it was also very painful, especially for Elizabeth, who is the eldest and the most affected by Chris' illness.

My children have been affected by having already lost their father and living with the fear that they might lose me. We don't talk about it a lot because it's a sore spot. Even little Christine knows about AIDS, although she doesn't know about HIV. She associates headaches with people that are dying from AIDS, because when her daddy was dying he had a severe headache from the meningitis. If I tell Christine that I have a headache she becomes very worried and fearful, and will fetch a towel to mop my forehead and tell me to take an aspirin. I don't know if this is because she believes that I might have AIDS. Certainly my other daughter, Betty (Elizabeth) fears that I might have AIDS. For children in a family where a member has any kind of terminal disease the anxiety is constant. But this is a part of life, isn't it? When you love someone you are always fearful that they will die. AIDS in one sense is just something to focus on. If it wasn't AIDS it would be something else. Every time I go away I fear that something will happen to my children. When I counsel people I tell them that they could be run over by a bus before they die of AIDS, but for children that's pretty hard to take.

Looking at Elizabeth I feel she has suffered on her own, alone. She didn't talk about it. Only once she talked about my involvement in TASO. She asked me, "Mummy, can't you find another job? Can't you find any other thing to do other than work in TASO?" She didn't seem to appreciate that for me this was a commitment, a dedication. She felt hurt that I worked with AIDS, and talked about her father dying. It hurt each time. Everytime she saw people with AIDS, when they came to the house, it brought memories back. She wouldn't join in any talk about AIDS. This situation is changing now, Elizabeth is talking a little more openly now.

Phiona reacted differently. She talks about AIDS and is involved in AIDS awareness at school. The children of Philly Lutaaya, the Ugandan singer who died of AIDS, are her friends, especially Tessa and Tina. They can sit down and talk about AIDS, especially Phiona and Tessa, Tina doesn't talk much.

In Uganda death and dying are issues very much with children. There are many orphans. They have lived with death and killing, first because of our political situation, now because of AIDS, and for many other reasons. My daughter Marion told me that virtually every week a child is collected from her boarding school because her mother is dying of AIDS, or has died in a car accident, or some other accident.

When I was young, if your father or mother annoyed you, or you felt more inclined towards one parent, you would sometimes ask how the world would be without that parent, what would happen if one parent died. For example, with mummy things might be easier because I could get whatever I want, that kind of thing. This question is no longer possible when one parent has died, because the next one to go will be the last. I sometimes sense this in my children, more so as they grow up. We have been talking increasingly about a house. They ask where they would be if I died. At least if we had a house they could stay in it whatever happened. If I died today my children would have to be split up to live with their father's brothers - unless we had a house they could continue to live in.

The concern for a house, a home, relates to a particular fear of being split up. Children belong to the husband's clan in our culture, so when one of my sisters-in-law died her husband's people came and took the children. In theory, if I died my children would have to go to my mother-in-law, who lives in a village. She already cares for 10 children, and she's old and heartbroken. She is a very hardworking woman, and has been growing her own food until this last year. She is now 64, and has lost three of her ten children to AIDS. She doesn't like to talk about it. The last three years have made a big difference to her. All she has left now is love, and she doesn't know how to share it. Her grandchildren remind her of the children she has lost, and my two girls have begun to sense that when their granny looks at them she remembers their father. It is difficult for her when she visits us because we talk about Christopher a lot. She either keeps quiet or changes the subject. Culturally we don't talk about the dead.

All my mother's children were still alive, until this year. My sister, Rose, who was only a year older than I am, became ill with AIDS, and died in May 1991. I now look after Rose's three children. My younger sister Harriet is also HIV infected, and is now ill with AIDS.

In my country and culture we talk about death, but not about the dead by name. We use different words to refer to them, for example the departed. There are a lot of different names for death. I felt it would be healthier for my children to think about their father in a more positive way. They know their father is dead, and the only way they will meet him again is by dying.

My mother-in-law doesn't want to talk about any of her children who have died, except in very rare circumstances. She has lost four children, three to AIDS, and it hurts her very much. My father-in-

> The other aspect which we address ourselves to, which is becoming an increasingly big aspect of the social welfare of AIDS, is the question of orphans. AIDS in Uganda, and in Africa in general, is affecting the young childbearing population. Where we have been able to reach out to people, and where they have been able to accept the final, the ultimate, consequence of HIV infection, the question that we are confronted with is "What about my children?". "What happens to my children in the event that I go?" This is also my own personal crusade, because I am a mother of four lovely daughters.
>
> My daughters! I keep saying to people, If I can contribute to a campaign which will succeed in keeping this age group free, a group (5-15 yearas old) which is emerging in Uganda statistics as not yet being affected, I will be happy.
>
> (Keynote Address to the Women and AIDS Support Network Conference, 23rd November 1989, p18).

law's attitude is different. Traditionally, I'm not supposed to be close to my father-in-law, but he's a more accepting person. When my sister-in-law was ill he was the one who sent her to me, who told her that she had to have the blood test. With him I could say, "I think she has AIDS". When she died my father-in-law said publicly, at the funeral, that she had died of AIDS. He talked of it as a terrible disease that had to be stopped, and one way to stop it was by being open about it. My sister-in-law had four children by different fathers I have never met. Settling the children is an important consideration on the death of a parent. Are they going to be looked after by their fathers, or are they are going to join the increasing group of orphans needing care?

In counselling parents who are elderly I am never sure of the value of telling them that their child has AIDS. Some people say it prepares them better, prepares them for any eventuality. I suppose it depends on the person. Should parents be told? I try to encourage people to identify one person they are close to and tell them. It then becomes a family responsibility to think about the parents, the spouse, etc. The only real reason for telling anyone about the AIDS diagnosis is positive living. If I judge the situation such that positive living is beyond reach, I don't see any reason to tell the parents about the cause of death. I would allow the parents to grieve for the person without adding the difficult cross of AIDS. It may be easier, for example, to publicly claim the body of a son who was a robber and thief, than one who had AIDS. They would come out more easily. The shame attached to death as a thief is less than that attached to AIDS. This is awful, and is now changing, but it is why you find people bending over backwards to call the illness all sorts of names other than AIDS. If a family needs that kind of protection they should have it. This, of course, has implications for death certificates, and what is written on them. In some circumstances it is justifiable to write that the person died of pneumonia or meningitis rather than AIDS, if this protects the privacy of the family. The statistics on AIDS can be collected from other more public data.

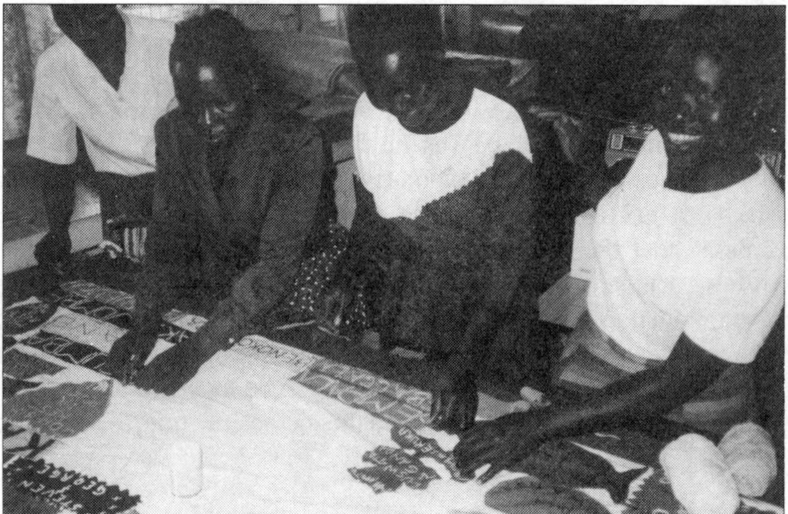

Making the TASO quilt with the names of those loved ones who have died

Living Positively With AIDS

The philosophy of 'Living Positively With AIDS' was adopted by the original TASO group for two main reasons.

First, at that time the public health messages were saying "Beware of AIDS, AIDS kills", "You catch it and you are as good as dead". There were no messages for those people who were already infected. What was implied was that people who were already infected should die and get it over with. People with HIV and AIDS were seen as dying. We adopted the slogan of "living positively with AIDS" in direct defiance of that perception. We emphasised *living* rather than *dying* with AIDS. For us it was the quality rather than quantity of life which was important. Once infected with a deadly virus like HIV people need to take definite steps to enhance the quality of whatever life they have left. They must develop a positive attitude to life.

Having a positive attitude means:

* knowing and accepting that they are infected
* knowing and understanding the facts about AIDS
* taking steps to protect others from their infection
* taking care not to expose themselves to further HIV infection or other infections
* taking special care of their physical health, and treating symptoms of ill health as soon as possible
* having access to emotional support
* continued participation in social life
* eating well and avoiding or learning to cope with stressful situations.

This seemingly complex philosophy is attainable. Achieving positive living is a process, with ups and downs, in which we all need support. It is part of working through the various feelings that having HIV may bring: shock, denial, anger, bargaining, acceptance and hope. Counsellors, carers, and friends, should learn to recognise this instability, and not be frustrated when progression through the stages seems erratic, and we regress to former emotional reactions. We need to be accompanied through these stages by a sensitive, understanding friend who pledges to be there for us.

The TASO slogan is "Living Positively with AIDS", and calls on everyone in society, infected or non infected. To the person who is infected it calls on them to live responsibly with the HIV infection in their blood, to face up to the infection as a starting point. It calls upon them to recognise their responsibility to society, the responsibility to retain the amount of virus they have in their blood, and not spread it around, by making the effort not to infect others. It also calls upon people who are infected to look after themselves better, and preserve themselves until a cure comes. It calls to people who are infected to remain actively involved in society, and in social activities within society.

It also calls upon the rest of society to support people with HIV infection so that they can fulfill their obligations. It calls on those who are not infected, or don't know whether they are infected, to accept people with AIDS, to recognise that you cannot catch AIDS through casual contact. Acceptance of people with HIV or AIDS within our community is a very important starting point for dealing with the problem.

AIDS affects ordinary people. AIDS does not affect the poor, does not affect the affluent. It affects a cross-section of people. AIDS effects you and me.

The starting point for living positively with AIDS, within our own bodies or within the family, is to know that we have AIDS. This information must be given accurately, consistently and sensitively. I believe that people must be told. First, they must know that they have been exposed, like I know that I have been exposed. Because of what I know about HIV infection I assume that I'm HIV infected, and whether the blood test is negative or positive I know that I have been exposed. That is the important thing to recognise. Whether someone is infected or not after they have been exposed to the virus, what is important is that they aren't exposed again, and that they don't expose others.

> Living positively with AIDS begins with the person getting to know the diagnosis. You can't begin to live positively if you do not know that you are HIV positive.

Living positively with AIDS begins with the person knowing, and as much as possible accepting, that they are HIV positive. They must then learn about AIDS, and expose themselves to information about the disease. Some people say "I don't want to hear anything about AIDS. I'm infected and that's enough".

We cannot live positively with AIDS if we don't know about it. There is a lot of stupid talk about AIDS which may be worrying for those who are positive but don't know enough about the infection. They put a question mark on themselves everytime anything is said. Stupid things, like catching AIDS through glasses or by sitting next to someone who is infected; or discussions about death and dying in which people predict death in two months, or three weeks, for those who are infected. If people with HIV don't have the information to check these myths against, it is difficult to live positively.

Soon after Chris died and I returned from the village, I started to eat obsessively because I was so stressed. I would eat anything I could lay my hands on and I became very fat. People started saying about me "You know with AIDS, if it's going to kill you it first fattens you, gradually you become fat and round, and within two months you start to become thin". Had I not known more about AIDS, that alone would have stressed me and would have caused me a lot of pain. When I checked this kind of information against that I knew scientifically, it didn't correlate. I knew I was getting fat because I was eating. So I knew that if I went off food I would lose weight.

> After Chris died I started to eat obsessively. I was reacting to stress, the stress of the stigma, the stress of having to live life without Chris. I was also pushed by the need to show people that I was not sick. I think I was deliberately eating to become fat. To be fat is to be fit and healthy, and I remember constantly, without having to think about it, needing to show that I wasn't fitting into my clothes anymore, that I had to buy new clothes.

With proper information people will not waste so much time and money going from one traditional healer to another, or from one physician to another, especially as some of them are unscrupulous. Some posh doctors, without the slightest conscience at all, will tell positive clients that they have typhoid, a disease which is rampant in Uganda and can easily be caught, especially in the cities, by drinking unboiled water. The doctors perpetuate the patients' visits to them in this way, and make a lot of money for themselves. The patients are themselves more comfortable with this diagnosis, and if the counsellor says anything different from the doctor the counsellor is the bad person - the AIDS prophet of doom. I remember when I first told a friend that I suspected that she was HIV infected, she was very annoyed and accused me of thinking that everyone had AIDS because my husband had died of AIDS. It wasn't fair, but she never came back to say, I'm sorry you were right.

People have to know the facts about transmission. Is it safe to hug their children? It is very painful for mothers who know they are HIV infected. They may stop holding their children for fear that they will infect them. This creates a point of agony. They may want to hug the children, to be near them, but, because they have the children's interests at heart, they remove them from their room.

Living positively with AIDS requires learning about AIDS, and coping with stress. This is one side of living positively. It is also very important to take definite steps not to infect others, and ensure that they are not exposed to further infection themselves. This needs to be explained quickly clearly to people with the infection. Many people think that once a person is infected with HIV they can't catch other infections or even add to the HIV infection they have.

Personal Victory over the Virus

It is important to impress upon people that if they don't pass the HIV infection on to any other person this would be their personal victory over the virus itself. The quantity of virus that they have in their blood cannot survive in any other way than to go into another person's blood. If they allow the virus to move out, they allow it to survive and prosper, even long after they die.

This is the only way the virus lives. We know that once the virus leaves the blood it is finished. The virus doesn't want to kill you, because the day it kills you it also dies. This is not in its own interest. It only intends to multiply, but in so doing it kills you. It is only while you remain alive that it can spread. The day you die the quantity of the virus that is in you is buried with you and is finished. When it infects you it destroys you, but without intending to do so.

We have very interesting sessions in the day centres in TASO putting this kind of scenario into plays. We have found that once people have understood the virus in this way, by using role plays, they can see that the virus can also be defeated. At that moment they know that they can't kill the virus, but it can be defeated by them.

For a person like me such a victory over the virus is only a partial victory. The virus has already killed my husband. The only way I can defeat it is by not allowing it to go into any other person.

Once people know that they are HIV infected they need to keep healthy, and one way to do this is by not ignoring symptoms of ill health. This does presuppose that people have access to care. It's pointless to talk about treating symptoms as they emerge if there's nowhere to turn to for treatment. This is one of the reasons why TASO also provides medical care.

People with HIV will be ill from time to time, and these illnesses are treatable. To be treated properly they have to be treated early. But where are people to go for treatment? In Uganda the situation is particularly difficult because the health service infrastructure was battered over 20 years of civil strife. Someone from my home village, for example, 40 kms from Kampala, who needs hospital care would have to catch a bus which comes only once a day, in the morning. This bus gets into Kampala around 10 am. The person would then proceed to Mulago Hospital and see the doctor. By about 3 pm the person will have seen the doctor and received a prescription. She will then take the prescription to the pharmacy window, where there will be another line of 100 people, and the window closes at 4,30. This means she has to come back the next day. If she has a relative in Kampala then she is lucky to have somewhere to stay. The following morning she lines up at the window again. The prescription is for four different medicines, but the hospital pharmacy has just one. So she takes that one and then rushes back home, if the one bus for that day has not yet left.

Another essential aspect of positive living is social life. It's very important to avoid isolating people with HIV. For instance, I don't know when I last went to a wedding. If a person is going to continue participating in social activities, society must accept it. If someone arrives at a wedding and everybody turns their heads to look at them, it is very uncomfortable. In TASO now we have our own weddings. In the day centres weddings are arranged for people who have been living together and want to get married. People have also been rebaptised, by a priest who comes to baptise them. These are big functions. They allow people to have some social interaction and to mark important life events.

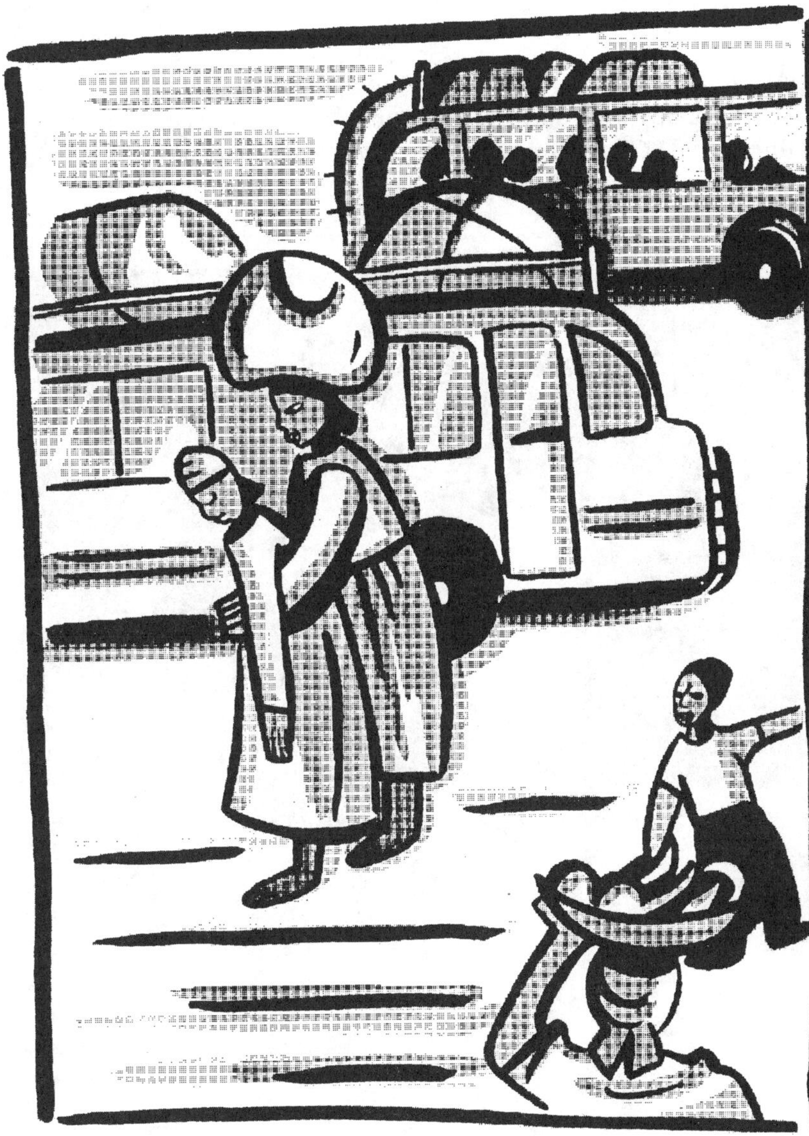

Another important celebration, held every year, is the birthday of TASO. This event also celebrates all those who are still alive at each birthday.

As more and more people are living with AIDS, the old fashioned feeling that if you have AIDS you are dead or dying should be thrown out. Given improved care, and a better understanding of the disease, people are living longer and better quality lives.

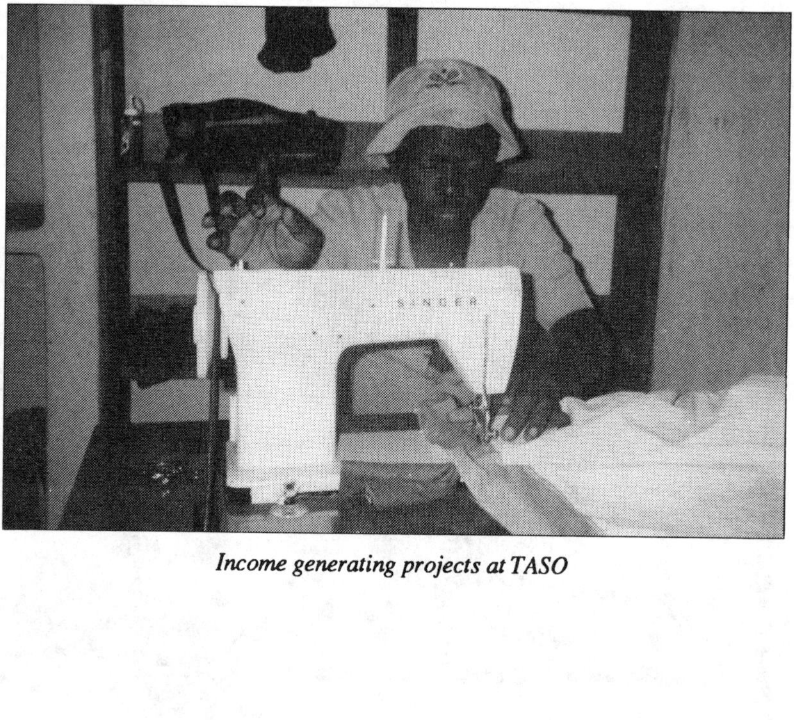

Income generating projects at TASO

Clinical Care

While AIDS care needs to be integrated into existing health and social services, we in TASO recognise that providing some specialised services, including clinical care, cannot be avoided. However, it is important to ensure that the emotional needs of people with HIV and AIDS are met along with health care.

In TASO outpatient clinical care is provided by committed doctors who have expressed an interest in working with AIDS. They are also trained in counselling so that they are more aware of the counselling issues and are able to highlight them when they refer patients for ongoing support and counselling. These doctors do not carry out the counselling in the clinic. It is important to recognise that the information provided to the patient by the doctor is consistent with that provided by the counsellor. Traditionally patients respect doctors, and believe what they say is important. The patient-doctor relationship is a powerful one. For this reason TASO impresses upon counsellors the importance of not misleading patients into thinking they are doctors. This can be done by constantly referring to the patients doctor in interviews, especially on issues of physical health. Clients know that the counsellors are not doctors, and if the doctor's and counsellor's information are different then the client may lose confidence in the counsellor, rather than the doctor.

Sensitivity to the role of the doctor may be particularly important when working with doctors who are 'traditionalists', who talk about 'my patient' and are resistant to sharing responsibility for the care of the patient. There are many doctors like this. Until all doctors, physicians and surgeons recognise that AIDS care is total care, involving not only the doctor, but also the family, the counsellor, and others, there will be a need for specialised AIDS clinics. For this reason every TASO facility runs a referral clinic once or twice a week. This requires a doctor, because in most cases the people TASO reaches are already ill with a physical complaint. It also requires a trained nurse. Once there is a doctor and a nurse, the counsellors could be teachers, housewives or others trained to provide this service.

After doctors make a clinical diagnosis, they tell the patients that the chances are very high that they are infected with HIV. The patient would have told the doctor that they have had a fever, a cough, a rash, whatever. They know these are the symptoms of AIDS. With these symptoms the chances are very strong that they are infected. A blood test could be made, and blood taken, but by the time the patients leave the doctor they have a clinical diagnosis, and they understand that the blood has been taken only to confirm the diagnosis.

In Uganda AIDS is a clinical diagnosis. A person who has AIDS doesn't have to have an HIV test before they are treated, because AIDS is a clinical manifestation. We are not treating HIV, we are treating the opportunistic infection. Do they have diarrhoea, do they have pneumonia, do they have TB, do they have typhoid? In Uganda, children born to people with HIV infection are not HIV tested until they are at least two years old, because a test done any earlier would not be conclusive, and would be a waste of resources. Children of HIV infected mothers are followed up to monitor their development.

When we started at TASO we did not register anyone that had not had a blood test. Now we register anyone with a clinical diagnosis, provided they have been diagnosed by a doctor we recognise and know. We tell them that one of the things they need to do immediately is to establish a support system and start to live positively.

Counselling at TASO

People with HIV must be informed about their infection in a sensitive consistent manner by someone who knows about HIV and AIDS and cares about people. They need to be helped through the typical shock reactions, and from shock to denial, anger, bargaining, acceptance and hope. They need to be accompanied through these stages by someone who recognises the inevitably of the stages. Someone who will accept and appreciate the anger, even if it is turned on them. Coping with this can be difficult, but has to be done. We have to find ways to help people open up, in creative ways, like using role plays. Otherwise a counsellor can become emotionally burnt out.

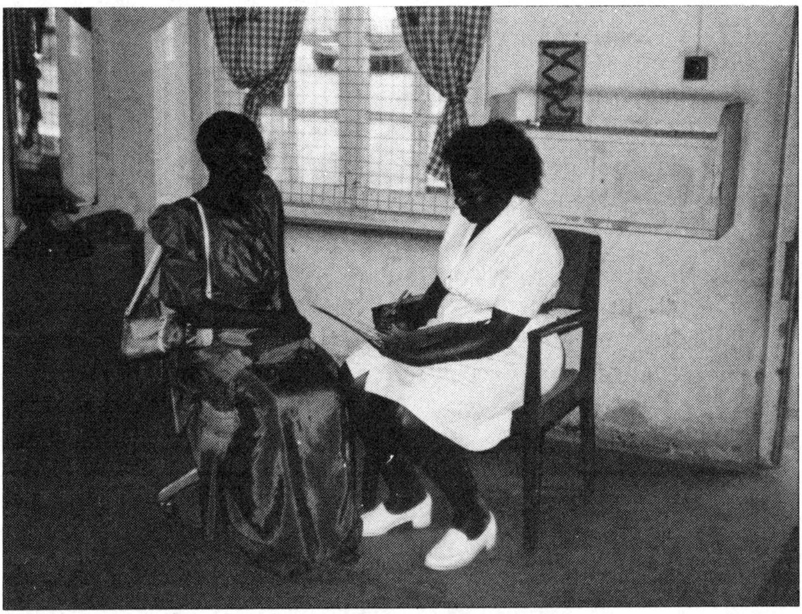

Jane in counselling with Noerine

Fortunately in TASO I don't have to do the counselling by myself anymore. We now have a large group of counsellors and other people with AIDS. It is an advantage in TASO that there are people with AIDS among the counsellors. Their participation is very important, although they have different levels of education and understanding. The group of counsellors meet regularly once a fortnight. I do everything possible not to miss these meetings. Because I have chosen to believe and to behave as if I am infected I am able to understand people with AIDS, empathise with them and live the life they live, at least emotionally. This attitude I feel has helped me in my work.

During the counselling meetings people can share their experiences on how to cope with particular problems. It's all so new that people are finding their own answers. They are drawing from inside themselves to work out ways of resolving a problem, or helping someone to resolve a problem. We all find the counselling meetings very useful. We don't deal with techniques but with major issues. We allow people to challenge each other, for example, if someone feels that other people are hindering their work. At the regular meetings everybody is encouraged to point out who is hindering their work. People are quite frank at the meetings, although some people take the criticism deeply, believing that others don't like them or blame them for not doing things.

However, as much as we value and explain the value of these meetings, there can be problems. One big problem for us was a division between the PWA counsellors (peer counsellors, people with AIDS) and what we call the 'anonymous'. The 'anons' are those who haven't been tested. The PWAs claimed that the anon group didn't, and couldn't, understand their situation. This was even carried through to clients, who were asked "Who is your counsellor? Oh, that one! They can't even begin to understand. They learnt their techniques in the classroom not from experience."

It was a bad time, but we had to face this division and deal with it. There were a lot of tears from the anon group who felt under a lot of pressure. It also seemed that they did not appreciate, despite their training, how to recognise different emotions. This is an important point. Those who wish to work with people with AIDS must recognise that the stages of shock, denial, forgiveness, anger, etc do not necessarily follow a neat and consistent pattern. For example, a client you felt you were doing well with, who appeared to have accepted things, suddenly appears with a newspaper report claiming that those with AB blood group cannot be HIV positive. The patients decide that they have been given the wrong results, it could not have been theirs, they don't have AIDS, because their blood group doesn't catch AIDS. The counsellor has to start from the beginning again. Counsellors should be able to understand why clients react like this, and deal with it. Dealing with AIDS is very frustrating work.

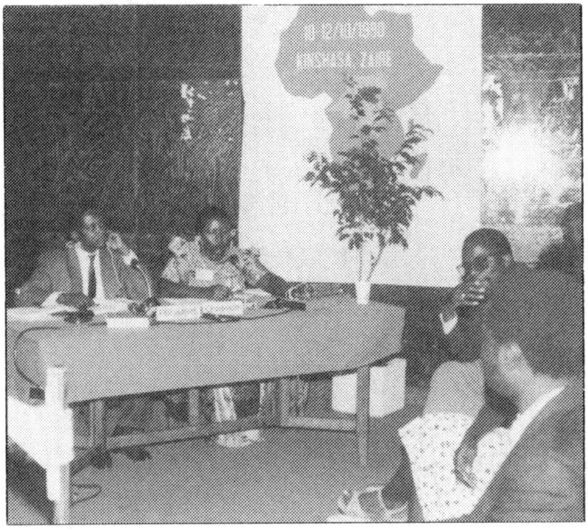

Home visit with a peer group counsellor

A good counsellor needs some basic knowledge. Good consistent counselling helps people recognise which symptoms are important and which are just anxiety, taking into account the personality of the person with AIDS, or without it. Some people are very anxious, they live in perpetual fear of illness. If they haven't gone to a medical centre for a week they must be dead!

In TASO's approach to HIV counselling and care, faith and religion are optional. Spiritual counselling is available, but everyone, whether they are Muslim, Christian, or atheist, should feel at home in TASO, feel they can come to us. In the original group that set up

TASO, most of us were practising Christians who would meet to pray together. We made a conscious decision to make TASO a non-religious organisation so that it would be open to everyone, that even non-religious people should find sustenance in it. I am a Catholic and my Christian faith has been a strong pillar of personal support for me. I can share this faith with clients if they want me to, but I keep it to myself unless I feel that the person in front of me is ready to share the Christ that I hold dear. I am very much opposed to people who present Christianity as a pre-requisite for help.

My Personal Support System

There are a number of factors in my life which have supported me in the fight against AIDS: faith, children and personal support from friends.

First, is *God, my constant faith in Him*, and the fact that He has loved me, and taken it upon Himself to give me continued life.

I was brought up as a Catholic by my mother, and even when I displeased her by marrying Chris, a non Catholic, I never stopped going to church. The children always went with Chris to the Protestant church because he insisted on this, and I went to the Catholic church. During the time he was in England we all went to the Catholic church.

From the time I received the telex from England, I prayed like I had never prayed before. I prayed for a miracle everynight. I prayed that I would get up in the morning and things would be different. I could not concentrate on normal routine prayers so I started talking to God directly, willing Him to change things. All this was done in tears, on my knees. I had found a new relationship with God.

I was not aware of this special personal relationship with God until I had this traumatic experience. I am always amazed that God loves me even as I am. I also know that to deal with a problem of the magnitude of AIDS, one has to have faith in some supernatural power. Those of us who have this experience of knowing God are very privileged, for we have something to relate to. This does not mean that people who do not know God are doomed. God in His infinite love will bring them friends, will act through children and relatives, and will make Himself known. This is why our acts of kindness should be universal and go across nations to all people. It is through our actions that His light will glow.

When traditional prayers failed me, I prayed through Our Lady and an uncannonised saint, Maria Theresa - but I also talked directly with

God. From that time I have shared my weaknesses with Him and asked Him for strength and direction each day. Right now I know the direction He is showing me is to reach out, with compassion, to people with AIDS. I also know He wants me to share my experience with others. This is where I derive the strength to stand up and talk about my experiences at conferences, on TV, at home, and at gatherings. He exposed me to suffering and stigma, and took my husband away as a process of preparing me to reach out. He loaned me life, children, and friends to equip me to meet the challenge, and made me articulate and able to understand. But He has not called upon me to preach the Gospel. I only share my faith with those clients who invite me to do so. I want His name to shine through my deeds.

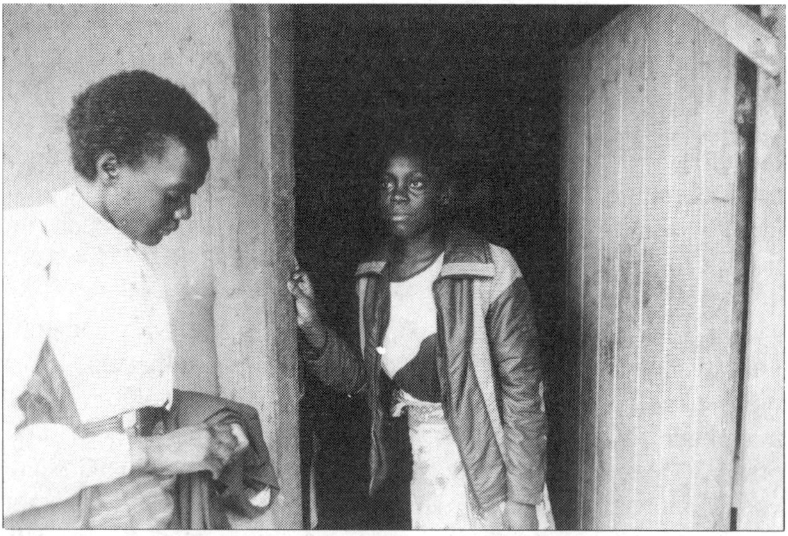

Noerine chairing a session on counselling

One aspect of my personal struggle is a God given gift, my attitude to life. This has always been positive, regardless of the circumstances. Faced with a problem I would always ask myself, is there anything I can do about it? Anything I can do to change this situation? If the answer was no, I would take steps to live with it and face up to it.

Second, is *my children*.

I don't know what I would have done without them. Their continued existence, and their continued good health, is part of my ongoing support. This was a very big factor for Chris too when he died. Every time I have faltered, every time I have felt the cross is too great to bear, I have thought about the children and how they are coping. I, at least, have been able to express my feelings and have been able to talk about AIDS openly. I have been able to ask many questions. My children, for the most part, have had to suffer silently - although there are times when I feel they are puzzling over issues and I have encouraged them to talk about them. Yes, my children are a big support, a big challenge, and a big reason to keep going.

Elizabeth Najjemba is 16 years old now and in her fourth year at Secondary School. She was our love child, born before our official marriage, but at the very peak of our love. She was well loved by Chris and his illness and death had a very definite effect on her. As she grows into a teenager she is having some problems. Talking to Betty you are always lecturing. She won't react, just sits and listens politely, but won't give feedback. I find this frustrating. She's a bit like Chris, he was very bright, but he didn't talk much, only to people he knew very well. She never talks about AIDS and does not come to TASO. Elizabeth is the one who has suffered the most from the illness and death of her father, and if she ever reads this account I want her to know that I love her dearly.

Phiona Nakalawa is 15 years old, our second born, born soon after our wedding. She is in her third year of secondary education. She is a sensitive girl and a born again Christian. I know she has met Christ because of the way she behaves. I pray that one day all her sisters will experience the joy and peace of mind which Phiona seems to radiate. She is very supportive of my work with TASO, but urges me to take it gently. Phiona is the family friend, and writes a letter to everybody once a month. I talk to her because she is a companion, she is the kind of girl who will come and start a conversation.

Marion Buzannyo, who is now eleven years old, is a sweet black beauty. She is everybody's favourite, and welcomes everybody with a hug. She is in her fifth year of primary education. She does not enjoy her life at school because she hates being away from home, although I think it is better for the children to be at boarding school when I am away from home so often.

Christine Nakiyemba is the very centre of our family. She is the baby, now seven years old and in her first year of primary education. She was only two and a half years old when her father died.

Third, is *the long line of friends* that God has brought in my path during this very difficult time.

These friends begin in the family, especially my in-laws. There is also my extended family in Britain. They were so compassionate and kind when TASO was formed, and some people have kept in close contact with me ever since, supporting the family in so many ways.

I would like to single out a few people, a few friends. People who, as soon as we knew that Chris was going to die, asked us how they could help. When we said we were worried about the children's education, they assured us they would help. The venture was spearheaded by Jan Webster, who I now look upon as a sister and who, I know, will always be there for me. These people probably don't want to be talked about, but they have really helped and supported me - Nadir Dinshaw, Harriet Gilmour, Patricia Chew, one of Chris's nurses, Reverend Father Storey, and the March's children, Judy and her special friend Paul. They are friends, they send presents, and they write letters of support which have helped to sustain us.

There are also the many friends who helped in so many ways as I started TASO. A very special category of friends, for whom I have very great respect, are my friends who have AIDS and HIV. Friends who were themselves ill when we met, but who agreed to participate

> In countries where there are increasing numbers of people falling ill with AIDS, it poses a big challenge to all of us who are talking about AIDS in whatever capacity. There are a lot of scientists working on research in AIDS and producing epidemiological data. There is a lot of talk about HIV and AIDS. People stand up at conferences and say what should be done, but a lot of this has not been translated into action. One very real way in which we can show action in AIDS is by caring and by offering support to people who are diagnosed positive, whether they are friends, people with AIDS, people with HIV infection, or their families. I have sat time and time again with elderly mothers and grandmothers whose talk of their dying loved ones has left an indelible mark upon my heart.

in this work, and who continued despite the suffering and pain, the stigma and ostracism. We stuck together and started the work of TASO.

Initially, when forming TASO, we met at my house, the Cheshire Home, or in my office at the School of Physiotherapy. One of the things I recall about this period was the encouragement given to me by George Makombe, one of the disabled people at Cheshire Homes, who is a close friend and who was a source of inspiration for me from the beginning.

I also count among my friends and as my support those who took the risk of supporting my programme in Uganda. I call it a risk because when we started this work we were seen as a group of lunatics talking about AIDS care. I had approached a few agencies prior to approaching Action Aid. Their reaction was very cautious. They were honest with me. They said that what I was proposing had not been done before, so they didn't have a model for comparison. Funding and support were, therefore, a risk which they were not prepared to take at that time. The long list of people who come to our support in the beginning, included Action Aid Director, Colin Williams, World in Need, and USAID. They came to our assistance as a result of one person from each organisation sitting down and listening to what we were saying.

Fourth, is the *opportunity for counselling myself.*

I only go to my counsellor when I have problems. I don't go for regular support. In this sense I have underutilised her. But she is very busy. The counsellor client ratio at TASO is one to 40, which is very big. She has to cope with that load and also do training. She has been a friend. She was my matron of honour when I got married, and is godmother to one of the children. She knows the family background and supported me when Chris was dying. She would spend a night in the hospital so I could go home to the children.

I do think people doing this kind of work need regular counselling, because issues turn up that you need to share with someone in a counselling situation. HIV counselling is not only to do with a person who is ill with AIDS, but has a lot to do with the emotions that arise from this. New situations constantly arise, even for me today the stigma doesn't seem to die. You know, sometimes you think that the situation is okay and then something will happen and all of a sudden you find yourself stigmatised in a completely different way to anything you had anticipated. Then you do need someone to talk to, someone to carry you through the emotions that arise.

Message for the Future

My message to all people in the world is one of hope. Hope for a future world without AIDS. This hope will come out of a realisation that the whole population, the infected, the affected and the uninfected, need to join the fight against AIDS. This hope also hinges on each one of us, as individuals, taking up the fight against AIDS. The responsibility to curb the spread of HIV lies with each person as an individual. Collective efforts by government and non government agencies relies on each individual's determination to refrain from the type of behaviour which puts them at risk of contracting HIV infection.

To everyone living with HIV infection or disease the message is of hope, and the courage to fight until a cure is found. We triumph over the virus when we do not allow it to spread! We do not, however, have to fight alone, in isolation. There are increasing numbers of friends willing to share with us and accompany us through this difficult period.

As Philly Lutaaya (RIP), who died of AIDS on the 15th December 1989, sings:

> In times of joy
> In times of sorrow
> Let's take a stand and fight on to the end
> With open hearts
> Let's stand up and speak out to the world
> We'll save lives
> Save the children of the world.

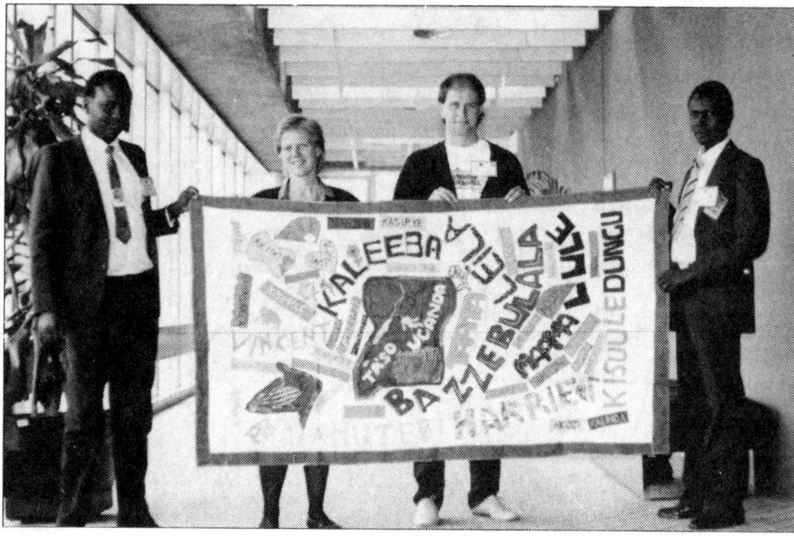

The first TASO quilt

The Names Project is an international project which commemorates the people whose lives have been affected by AIDS. Relatives, partners and friends have sewn panels with the names of their loved ones and some symbols of their lives. These panels are then joined together to make one enormous quilt which symbolises the grief and love felt by all these people for those who have died. It also makes a statement that their lives are important and that they are deeply missed.

The originalTASO quilt was the first African panel to be included. The title for this book, **We Miss You All**, was drawn from the second TASO quilt (shown on the front page). The courage of the families who have put the names of their loves ones on the quilts have contributed towards a more open and supportive attitude towards people with AIDS.

Alone

Philly Bongole Lutaaya

Out there somewhere
Alone and frightened
Of the darkness
The days are long
Life is hiding, no more making new contacts
No more loving arms
Thrown around my neck.

Take my hand now
I am tired and lonely
Give me love, Give me hope
Don't dessert me, Don't reject me
All I need is love
And understanding.

Chorus:
Today it's me
Tomorrow someone else
It's you and me
We've got to stand up and fight
We'll shed a light in the fight against AIDS
Let's come on out
Let's stand together, fight AIDS.

In times of joy, In times of sorrow
Let's take a stand and fight on to the end
With open heart, Let's stand up and speak out to the world
We'll save some lives
Save the children of the world.

Let's be open
Advise the young ones
A new generation
To protect and love
Hear them singing
Playing, laughing
Let's give them everything
In truth and love
Take the message
Across the frontiers
Break the barriers
We'll fight together
The doors are open
We'll lead the struggle
We won't lie down in defeat
We'll fight on.

Chorus:

References

Society for Women and AIDS in Africa (SWAA) (1990) **Keynote Address**, Second Workshop on Women and AIDS in Africa, Lagos, Nigeria, 28th-31st May 1990.

The Herald (1990) Zimbabwe Newspapers, Harare, 18th October 1990.

Women and AIDS Support Network (WASN) (1989) **AIDS. An Issue for Every Woman**, Report of the First Conference, Harare, Zimbabwe, 23rd November 1989, 18.

Note:

Living Positively With AIDS: The AIDS Support Organisation (TASO), Uganda, by Janie Hampton, No 2 in the Strategies for Hope Series, is booklet which discusses the formation and growth of TASO. There are also two 20 minute video programmes which focus on the work of TASO.

For futher information about this booklet and these videos contact:

TALC
P O Box 49
St Albans
Herts AL1 4AX
UK.